EAT TO TRIM

EAT TO TRIM

GET IT OFF AND KEEP IT OFF!

JOYCE L. VEDRAL, PH.D.

WARNER BOOKS

A Time Warner Company

CREDITS
Bodywear provided by Dance France, 1-800-421-1543
Photography by Don Banks
Hair and makeup by Darienne Bramberg
Gym shoes by Reebok International

Nutritional information provided by Tiffany Middendorf, R. D., Nutritionist at the Pritikin Longevity Center, Miami Beach, Florida. Nutritional analysis of recipes generated by Manage Your Diet program, Cynergy Marketing, Inc. Additional information compiled from *Food Values of Portions Commonly Used* by Jean A. T. Pennington, Harper and Row, New York, 1989.

Warner Books, Inc., 1271 Avenue of the Americas, New York, NY 10020

A Time Warner Company

Printed in the United States of America
First Printing: January 1997
10 9 8 7 6 5 4 3 2 1

Library of Congress Cataloging-in-Publication Data

Vedral, Joyce L.
    Eat to trim : get it off and keep it off / Joyce L. Vedral.
        p.   cm.
    Includes index.
    ISBN 0-446-51887-5
    1. Reducing diets.   2. Low-fat diet.   I. Title.
RM222.2.V43   1997
613.2'5—dc20
                                        96-22082
                                         CIP

Book design by L&G McRee

*To all of the women (and men, too) who want to eat plenty
and stay slim and trim*

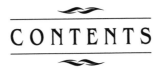

CONTENTS

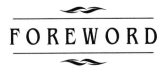

FOREWORD

Dieting in this country has become our national pastime. In fact, there are 50 million Americans currently on a diet. But according to a survey by *Consumer Reports*, 95 percent of the people who lose weight gain it all back within two years. Many dieters believe that they are failures, lacking the willpower and motivation to successfully lose weight and keep it off. The dieter is not at fault; however, the diet is.

Most diets put far too much emphasis on severe calorie restrictions, leaving you feeling hungry and deprived, so that the body actually slows down its calorie-burning machinery to ensure survival and develops an increased desire for fatty foods. This explains why dieters often end up eating far worse after the diet than beforehand.

The key to a successful weight-loss program is to consume an adequate number of calories to prevent this starvation response from triggering your fat tooth. *Eat to Trim* takes into account the negative consequences of stringent dieting. This food plan allows you to eat an abundance of nutritious and delicious food that promotes optimal weight loss without feeling hungry or deprived. The emphasis is not on severe calorie restriction, but on healthy, low-fat foods and frequent eating. Three meals and two snacks daily are an effective strategy to keep hunger at bay. This method of eating also stimulates the body's metabolism to burn more calories and promote easier weight loss. Combining the right proportions of carbohydrate, protein, fat, fiber, vitamins, minerals, and fluid results in an optimal way of eating for peak performance and ideal weight loss.

Eat to Trim will provide a wealth of information for the health-conscious individual. Not only does Joyce teach you all of the basic rules for eating a balanced, low-fat diet, she spells them out for you with 31 breakfasts, lunches, dinners, and 62 snacks. But it doesn't end there. All of the work has been done for you, which means no calculating and no guesswork.

Joyce worked diligently to develop meals with optimal amounts of carbohydrate, fiber, and protein while monitoring the overall fat, cholesterol, and sodium content. Many of her plans also include "quickie" meals, taking only a few minutes to prepare. Joyce's recipes for muffins, pancakes, soup, stews, vegetable combinations, and desserts are so flavorful, your concept of diet food will be forever changed. Chapter 9, "Meal Plans," will be your guide to achieving the ideal food plan for maximum weight loss.

Joyce also provides you with an inside look at her own personal weight-loss history, as a testament to the success she has had following this program. You will be inspired by the before and after photographs of men and women who have followed this program with wonderful success. They will help give you that extra boost of encouragement to meet your own personal fitness potential.

Best of health!
TIFFANY MIDDENDORF, R. D.
Senior Nutritionist, Pritikin Longevity Center

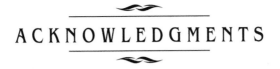

ACKNOWLEDGMENTS

To Joann Davis, for your continual support and enthusiasm.

To Mel Berger, my agent, for giving me the title for this book.

To Caryn Karmatz, for your kind willingness to go the extra mile.

To Flag, Diane Luger, and Jacki Merri Meyer, for your dedication to the cover art.

To Larry Kirshbaum, Mel Parker, and Emi Battaglia, for being every author's dream when it comes to backing me up.

To Don Banks, for your artistic photography.

To Dance France, for providing all of the workout clothing.

To Family Fitness Centers in Las Vegas, Nevada, and all over the United States, for providing a wonderful workout environment—and to Brad Marlow and David Bedwell, managers, and to Dominic Perez, assistant manager.

To Mike Kibler, for creating kitchens that motivate people to cook! And to Pat Lotta, his amazing assistant.

To Tiffany Middendorf, nutritionist extraordinaire—for your

endless patience in figuring the nutritional calculations—for your amazing expertise and good-natured sense of humor through it all! Bless you. A million times, bless you.

To family and friends, for your continual support.

To you, the women and men who have written to me requesting such a book.

EAT TO TRIM

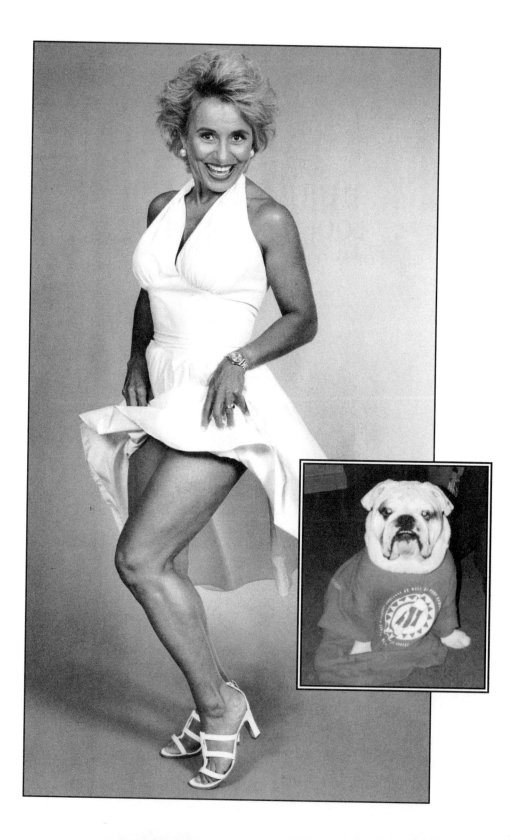

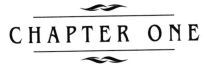

CHAPTER ONE

EAT LIKE A DOG, LOOK LIKE A DIVA
For People Who Love Food

I love to watch a hungry dog eat. You put the food in his bowl and a minute later it's gone. In fact, at times, I remind myself of a dog. I even wish l had a long snout like a dog so I could put my face in the plate and snap up the food even more quickly!

Yes, the truth is, if no one is around, and often even if they are, I can have a whole dish of food in front of me, and in a matter of minutes the food is gone. I've lost some future dates this way, I'm sure.

But the analogy between myself and a dog doesn't stop there. Like a dog, I like to eat more than a modest portion of food. In fact, if you turn me loose around food I love, I'll eat until I can't move. I'll talk more about where I learned these habits in Chapter 2, but for now suffice it to say that at times I still eat like a dog. Only now I eat foods that won't make me fat. In fact, that's why I invented this diet or, to put it in a less threatening way, this eating plan. Let's face it: what you eat on

1

a daily basis is your diet—at least that's what the dictionary says when you look up the word *diet*.

WHO ARE THEY KIDDING WITH THOSE TINY PORTIONS?

It always amazes me to see what recipe writers dare to call a portion. I can tell you straight out that it isn't unusual for me to eat at least two-thirds of an entire recipe that claims to serve four.

I'm not going to insult you. Most of the portions are larger than usual, yet you'll still lose weight. Why? Because the meal plans will still be low in fat and calories. Actually, the portions aren't *that* large—just a little larger than usual. And some recipes have no portion limits at all. These are your unlimited complex carbohydrates, and you can really go to town.

But what if these portions are too much for you and you don't want to eat that much? Great. You can cut them down to size. As long as you get your minimum nutrition in balance (and you will because I give you clear guidelines in Chapter 3) you'll be fine. But if you're like me, large portions will be the least of your worries.

EAT LIKE A DOG AND LOOK LIKE A DIVA: LOSE WEIGHT AND STILL ENJOY YOUR LIFE AND YOUR FOOD

So you love to eat but you don't want to look like Dave, my English bulldog, who at 69 pounds (mysteriously he has stayed that weight for years, no matter what he eats) looks like a fat white sausage. No, you want to look like a sexy goddess, a diva. (If you're a male reader, replace *diva* with *stud*.) Well, good news. You can do it. I show you how.

There will be no hunger pangs with this eating plan. You are required to put food in your mouth at least five times a day. (Occasional lapses are okay.) And what you eat will be surprisingly filling, delicious, and energizing. In addition, you can eat certain foods any time of the day. In other words, there will never be a time when you are hungry but will have used up your food allotment. Regardless of how much you've already consumed, there will always be the "free unlimited complex carbohydrates," as explained in Chapter 3.

This diet is in agreement with a low-fat version of the USDA's Food Pyramid. It is carefully formulated so you eat a nutritionally balanced menu on a daily basis while at the same time keeping your fat grams low. Women are allowed 20 to 25 fat grams a day (though some meal plans allow as low as 10 percent of the day's caloric intake, the minimum needed for good health), while men are allowed 30 to 40 fat grams a day.

If you follow this eating plan, you will get the right amount of low-fat protein, high-energy complex carbohydrates (starches and vegetables), healthful simple carbohydrates (fruit), and fat. Fat? Yes, I said fat. You can't totally avoid fat. You need some of it for good health and to prevent a feeling of continual hunger—a feeling that can force you to abandon good eating habits and binge like a madman.

Perhaps the best part of this diet is that it will benefit both your health and your vanity. Not only will you be regularly consuming ideal proportions of the various food elements for good health (prevention of cancer, heart disease, and other maladies), but you will at the same time lose excess body fat so that your body will be more appealing to the eye and the touch—and you'll have more energy, too! The end result will be that you will look and feel younger, and you may even extend your life.

WHY I WROTE THIS BOOK

Some of you may know me. I'm the author of several bestselling workout books (see Bibliography). While each of these books emphasizes exercise, I always include a chapter on eating. Without a proper diet, the perfectly formed, tight, defined muscles obtained through the workout would be covered with excess fat. In the diet chapters of these books, I present low-fat eating plans and up to a week's worth of meal plans. These meal plans were, I must admit, a bit boring and repetitive. Over the years, I received thousands of letters from my fitness readers: "Dr. Vedral, please, we're tired of those few meal plans you present. Can't you write a whole book about diet, and give us some recipes and a month's worth of motivating meal plans?" Well, the time has come, and here it is.

But you don't have to be a reader of one of my fitness books to take advantage of this weight-loss plan. In fact, if you are a new reader, this is a great way to become acquainted with my workouts. I've included a chapter on exercise here, because without exercise it's difficult to keep the weight off and impossible for your muscles to be tight and toned. With diet alone, you could end up as "skinny fat" at best.

BUT WHY SHOULD I DIET? IT'S NOT WHAT'S ON THE OUTSIDE THAT COUNTS

Famous words. We've all heard them, time and again. And no one believes these words more than I do. Beauty will fade. The body will eventually grow old and die. It's the soul that counts: what kind of a person we are and what we do with our life. Right?

Absolutely right. But here's the catch. If we don't pay attention to what's on the outside—the way our bodies look—we can be greatly hindered in giving what's on the inside to the world. It's difficult to use our creative energy to its fullest potential when we are always thinking, "I'm so fat, I'm so ashamed, I hate my body, I wish I could lose weight." And what makes it even more difficult is, like it or not, people react to us based on what they see.

When people first meet us, it's our body and not our soul that they see. If we could walk around town without a body— if people could immediately see our wonderful souls and never even glimpse our bodies—we could put the whole issue to rest right now and forget about our bodies. But the fact is, whether fair or not, the first thing people react to is our bodies. I don't like it any more than you do, but it's true.

If we are fat and unsightly, people often put up an initial barrier that we then have to work to break down. This would be okay if we were up to the task of breaking down that barrier, even if it did use up creative energy that could be better spent on other things. But the problem is, we are often not up to the job of dealing with the prejudice that people have to an unsightly body. Instead, we feel guilty and ashamed of ourselves.

We shouldn't feel guilty about or ashamed of our bodies. But it doesn't matter a whit that we *shouldn't* feel guilty or ashamed of our bodies. What matters is that we do. The end result is that the whole thing becomes too much for us—the barriers, the effort to break them down, and the guilt and shame we feel when trying to be charming, loving, and accepted. Having invested all that energy in trying to be accepted in spite of our bodies, we are too exhausted to use our energy creatively—doing what we were put on this earth to do, using our talents and abilities to the fullest. Instead, we obsess about our bodies, thinking about how to get the excess weight off, how to get people to love and accept us, how to find people who will not judge us by body image, and on and on.

I say, let's call the whole thing off. Instead of wasting precious time and energy on the overweight thing, let's get the weight off and get it out of the way. If we do that, not only will we be able to focus on what really counts, but we'll be able to do it in good health—and we'll probably live longer.

STARVATION DIETS MAKE YOU FATTER IN THE LONG RUN

Sure, you can go on a very low-calorie diet (under 1,000) and lose weight fast. But in the long run, your metabolism will slow down so that it is even harder to lose weight the next time you diet.

A recent study done with laboratory rats proves this point. Very fat rats were put on a starvation diet, and they lost all their excess weight in twenty-one days. Then they were allowed to eat as they pleased, and they quickly regained that weight. Before they could get any fatter (that is, the moment they were exactly the weight they started out with, their original fat weight), they were again put on the same starvation diet. This time it took them forty-two days to lose the weight—*exactly double the time.*

What happened? The rats' metabolism had slowed down. And it's the same with people. When you starve yourself, your body burns muscle, and it is muscle that keeps your metabolism burning fat (muscle is the only body material that burns fat twenty-four hours a day). In addition, your body goes into a survival mode and learns to conserve its food stores. In other words, your body slows down its own metabolism by burning its food stores (fat and calories) more slowly.

But, thankfully, if this has already happened to you, you don't have to worry. The problem is easily remedied by working out properly with weights—and I'm not talking about *heavy* weights. I tell you exactly what to do in Chapter 10.

HOW THIS EATING PLAN WORKS

Most people would like to eat what they want, when they want, and in the quantities they want, but they can't find a way to do it and not get fat. While you're losing weight, this eating plan will allow you to take advantage of the second two elements: eat *when* you want and *how much* you want. To eat *what* you want, you'll have to wait until you're at your fitness goal—and then you'll be able to do it in moderation either once a day—or in larger quantities once a week. I'll explain this on pages 82 to 84.

EATING OFTEN IS THE KEY

Ah, there is a catch. I'm not going to let you eat as much as you want unless you eat often. Yes. It has been proved that eating often will cause you to lose more weight. Since you are not forcing your body to go long periods without food, it doesn't feel starved, and when you do eat, you don't "shovel in" as much. In addition, when you are very hungry, you tend to reach for fatty, sugary foods, in spite of your best intentions. This is a starvation reflex, a survival instinct. Your body wants to get the most calories and energy it can quickly because it fears death. Did you ever notice that the times you break your diet are on days when you've starved yourself?

But there's another, even more important reason for eating at least five times a day. When you don't eat for more than five hours, your survival system kicks in in yet another way. Your metabolism slows down to a crawl, and you burn far fewer calories than you would have had you eaten at least a little food—a slice of whole wheat bread, some vegetables, a piece of fruit. For these reasons, this diet plan asks you to eat five times a day (more is optional). You will have three meals and two snacks, but your overall fat and calorie intake will be low enough to cause you to lose weight steadily. The best part is that your body will not fight you and try to gain the pounds back the minute you are off guard, because this eating plan is perfectly balanced nutritionally. Your body will be happy and content, rather than vigilant to enact the starvation response. It's the only way to lose weight and keep it off.

THERE ARE NO SHORTCUTS

A few years ago I was offered a large sum of money to allow a company to put my name on a liquid diet. In presenting their argument to me, the company said, "They'll lose weight—and that's what they want, so you'll be helping people."

Needless to say, I turned them down cold. Lose weight, indeed. But what happens after that? I know all too well that even those plans that allow the dieter to eat one "food" meal a day cause a retaliation effect once the liquid diet is stopped.

The only way to lose weight and keep it off is to follow a nutritionally balanced eating plan that will allow the body to comfortably let go of excess fat in a reasonable time, so that the body does not feel threatened and does not have the need to gain weight back.

Any diet that deprives the body of needed food substances will in the end backfire. It will force the body to overcompensate and binge on that food element that was deprived. Extreme low-carbohydrate diets are a prime example of this. I talk about this and other "quick-fix" diets in Chapter 2. The safest and most intelligent way to weight loss is to cooperate with Mother Nature.

HOW FAST WILL YOU LOSE WEIGHT?

I know. You want to lose it fast! Ten pounds a week would suit you just fine, but the truth is, the human body does not like to lose weight that fast. In fact, we don't even *gain* 10 pounds a week (or 520 pounds a year) even if we're eating with a vengeance night and day. Nor do we gain an average of 2 pounds a week. But the good news is, if you are significantly overweight, your body will allow you to lose an average of 1½ to 2 pounds a week. It will cooperate with you because it aims toward health and survival.

Of course you could "force" your body to lose faster by using fad diets, but as mentioned earlier, with those diets, the body eventually rebels and sooner or later (and it's usually sooner) you gain the weight back with some extra in the bargain. Eat to Trim is the opposite of such a plan. Instead of forcing your body to do something that is unnatural, this plan cooperates with your body by giving it the food it needs to operate at maximum capacity—and at the same time gradually shed all of your excess body fat.

You will lose weight gradually and surely—1½ to 2 pounds a week. When you get closer to your goal, your body will not be as eager to lose weight, and you'll lose more slowly. For instance, if you're 50 pounds overweight, you can count on the average of 1½ to 2 pounds of weight loss a week. But when you're only 20 pounds overweight, you may lose an average of 1 to 1½ pounds a week. When you're 10 pounds overweight, you'll lose only about ½ to 1 pound a week.

What happens when you're only 5 pounds overweight? I'll use myself as an example. I'm lucky to lose ¼ pound a week—being very strict. But I don't care. I just keep at it until I reach my goal. Why does it take so long when we're so close to the goal? The body would really love to keep those extra few pounds. It's the survival instinct of the body—a throwback to the caveman days when food may not have been readily available for a few days. But don't worry. With persistence and patience you can get rid of those last few pounds.

Also keep in mind that your body has its own losing pace. Some weeks you will lose weight and other weeks, even though you adhered strictly to the plan, the scale will stay the same or even go up (you may be retaining water). Don't be alarmed. Just stick to it and over the month, you will lose an average of 6 to 8 pounds of fat.

And don't "worry" that scale to death. Whatever you do, don't weigh yourself every day because water weight shifts depending upon what you've eaten (especially salt). You can weigh yourself once a week, but think more in terms of average monthly weight loss. In other words, at the end of the month, how much have you lost? And even better, see how much you lost after six months, then average it out on a monthly basis.

I'm giving you a relaxed way to think of losing weight. Why? It's the only way you'll keep it off. I've tried so many other diets, but this kind of dieting is the only way that works for me

and for the million or more women (and men too) who follow
my fitness books.

THE USDA's FOOD PYRAMID
AS A BASIS FOR THIS DIET

The USDA's Food Pyramid is a well-researched guide for getting the appropriate nutritional balance of foods in a given day.
It encourages consumption of large amounts of vegetables, an
ample amount of fruit, a generous supply of starches (filling
complex carbohydrates such as pastas, grains, breads, and
potatoes), a sufficient amount of dairy products, and a healthy
amount of protein. *Note:* If you have a problem with dairy
products, with your doctor's permission you can eliminate
them.

The difference between the diet presented in this book and
that of the USDA's guidelines is that you eat more vegetables
and I spell out specifically how much fat you are allowed to
consume. In addition, I give you lists of specific foods in each
category so you can stick to the most nutritious, low-fat foods
and lose weight faster.

Do you have to count calories? No. I count them for you,
although you can add them up if you want to, since they are
listed for your information at the end of each recipe and in all
the meal plans. More about calories in Chapter 3.

CHANGE YOUR MINDSET

Perhaps the most important thing about developing good eating habits is that it's not a temporary thing. In other words,
catch yourself when you start thinking, "I can't wait until I lose
this weight so I can eat again" (meaning, "go back to my old
eating habits"). Instead think, "I can't wait until my body gets
used to eating healthy and I no longer crave artery-clogging,

blubber-producing foods!" If you want rewards, think about the one day a week you will be able to eat "forbidden" foods—once you reach your goal and know that these foods will no longer be an issue for you.

FROM "EAT TO GRIM" TO "EAT TO TRIM"

As a child I was underweight. Once I got married, I gained 10 pounds every year until I began to look like my "box on wheels" Russian grandmother, my aunts, and my mother. I hated myself. I hated my life. I felt guilty every time I put food in my mouth. Though I talk more about this in Chapter 2, for now suffice it to say that I knew something was wrong. After a long, hard search, I discovered the secrets of permanent weight loss and have since shared them with thousands of women and men. Like me, they can now "eat to trim" instead of "eat to grim" and defeat. I want to share my secrets with you so you too no longer have to feel guilty every time you put food in your mouth.

WHAT YOU WILL FIND IN THIS BOOK

Before you get started, here's a quick overview of what you will find in this book.

Chapter 2: I tell you about my own fearful battle with food and how I discovered the right way to eat and lose weight. I talk about the psychological aspects of weight loss, and show you how to use mind power to gain control over food so that it is no longer a threat. I show you how to think of your diet as an "in training" positive rather than a punishment. Finally, you learn how the "free eating day" once a week works to keep you slim and happy.

Chapter 3: I present the basic nutritional facts, and simplify the whole issue of fat grams versus percentage of fat. I show you how to figure out your daily fat intake without being a mathematician. I talk about various types of fats, including the dangers of the so-called good fats, and explain how much of the nonfat foods you can *really* eat without getting fat. I deal with the complicated issues of vitamins, food supplements, caffeine, and alcohol. And I lay out my basic eating plan, or diet, and show you how to eat until you are stuffed and still lose weight on those days when you can't stop eating.

Chapter 4: I explain various nonfat cooking methods, and give special "get the fat out" food preparation techniques. I tell you how to use the exact spice for which foods for best flavor bursts, and talk about the few basic "cooking without fat" items you will need. I tell you what is actually in my refrigerator and food cabinets, and suggest brand-name food items such as pasta, rice, sauces, and soups.

Chapter 5: I offer you a whole month's worth of easy-to-prepare low-fat breakfasts, including ten quick-start breakfasts and an additional ten running "out of the house late" emergency breakfasts.

Chapter 6: I present a month's worth of easy-to-prepare low-fat lunches, including ten quickie lunches for those who are too busy to spend even ten minutes cooking.

Chapter 7: I give a month's worth of low-fat dinners that are simple to prepare, including ten quickie dinners that are amazingly delicious yet take only minutes to fix.

Chapter 8: I suggest a month's worth of low-fat snacks, including twenty quickie snacks that take less than a minute to make.

Chapter 9: I pull the eating plan together for you by supplying a month's worth of daily meal plans, using the food offerings in Chapters 5 through 8, so that you will not have to think. I include figures on total calories, protein, fat, sodium, and cholesterol. I also tell you how to keep to your diet when dining out. I talk about dealing with dieting while having to cook for a family, and explain how to work around a limited financial situation.

Chapter 10: This is the exercise chapter. Here, I explain why a little of the right exercise can up your metabolism so you can eat more without getting fat. I give a simple exercise plan (with photographs) that will tighten, tone, and shape your body. In addition, I explain which of my exercise books would suit your needs best, should you choose to go further with exercise.

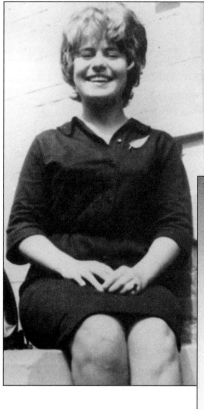

Joyce Vedral, 25
Before

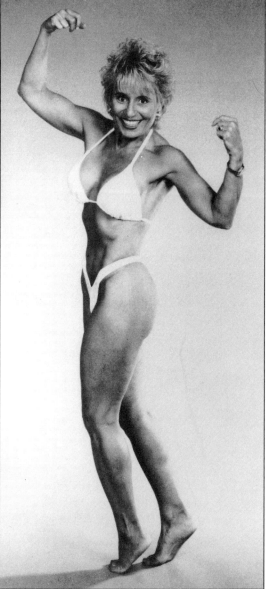

Joyce Vedral, 53
After

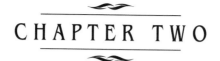

CHAPTER TWO

HOW I OVERCAME BEING CONTROLLED BY FOOD— AND HOW YOU CAN, TOO

It pains me to remember how it felt—how even in my twenties, I would see the rolls of fat on my stomach and back getting thicker and thicker. I would look at those rolls and vow to stop eating, only to eat twice as much that day. I would stuff myself until I literally felt as if I would burst, especially when no one was at home to see me. I recall with pain the guilt, the hopelessness I would feel afterwards. "Everyone in my family is fat. Why did I dream that I could escape that fate?" I would think.

Yes, it pains me to remember the shame I felt even when going to the doctor for a routine checkup, knowing that he might comment on how fat I was getting (and he did, and I hated him for it). But perhaps I can give you courage by showing you where I came from and where I am today. Perhaps I can help you to see that, even though our situations may be different, if I lost weight, you can, too.

FROM UNDERWEIGHT TO BUTTERBALL

I was a skinny child, underweight. I ate and ate and couldn't gain weight. By today's standards I would have been considered lean but healthy, but in the forties and fifties, I was viewed as undernourished and in danger of all kinds of diseases.

But I didn't stay skinny. I'm five feet tall, and when I got married at age 23, I weighed 98 pounds and wasn't underweight. I looked just right. But I didn't stay that way. I gained 10 pounds a year until I was in the "130s." I went from a size 3 to a size 13–15. I found myself in Weight Watchers, where I watched the scale every day in dread of that weekly weigh-in. And if I saw that the scale didn't go down that week, I took laxatives and diarrhetics. Hey, I wasn't going to let that scale beat me.

DIETS THAT DIDN'T WORK

Well, I did lose weight on Weight Watchers; in fact, Weight Watchers involves an excellent, well-balanced diet. I went down to 103 pounds. But frankly, I hated measuring and weighing, and monitoring myself, and I hated the scale. I became obsessed with it. It became my enemy. I hated the scale all the more when I finally reached my weight goal because, when I did, I was sadly disappointed. My body was droopy and saggy, and I didn't have a good shape. (I later found out that the sag was because I needed to work out with weights. More about this in Chapter 10.)

I eventually gained the weight back, and at 130-something, I ended up returning to meetings to re-lose the weight. After five or six rounds with Weight Watchers, I tried other diets.

My next attempt was a popular low-carbohydrate, high-protein, high-fat diet that allowed all kinds of fatty protein, including red meats, and hardly any carbohydrates. After two weeks of that diet, I lost 10 pounds. Even though I was so irritable that the diet cost me some friends and I couldn't concentrate enough to read a book, I didn't care. I was thrilled.

But my joy was short-lived. After five days off the diet, I gained back the whole 10 pounds. Two days later, I was 2 pounds heavier! In addition, I noticed that my body felt flabbier than before, even more droopy than when I was my fattest. And another thing happened. I couldn't stop eating: cookies, doughnuts, candy, cake—things I never craved before. One week later, I had gained another 3 pounds.

Now, in less than two weeks after I stopped the diet, I was 5 pounds heavier than I was in the first place. This depressed me and I really went to town and ate, until in about three weeks I had gained another 5 pounds. I was fatter than ever—142. I can remember to this day how I reset the scale down by 3 pounds so it would be 139. In fact, I brainwashed myself to believe that I never went over 130-something. But I remember my self-deception. Why not admit it now? I was 142 and gaining.

I later found out why, while on the diet, I was grouchy and irritable, and couldn't concentrate, why I had lost muscle tone and in the end was more droopy than I had been at the start, and why I not only quickly regained the lost weight with additional fat weight—and kept gaining fat weight:

1. Carbohydrates are the main supply for the brain's energy. Without an adequate supply of carbohydrates, I became irritable and couldn't even think straight. I had developed *phosphorous jitters*, a condition caused by excessive protein intake at the expense of carbohydrates. It comes about because of the high phosphorous but low calcium content of protein. The end result is a nervous, irritable temperament that is ready to snap at the slightest provocation.

2. I felt weak because it is carbohydrates that supply the body with energy.

3. I became flabby because I had deprived my body of carbohydrates. In the absence of carbohydrates, my body had used muscle for fuel—it began to literally eat itself. Once the diet was over, I had lost muscle, not fat. Of course, my body felt flabbier than ever.

4. The big amount of weight I lost in the beginning came back only a few days after I began eating carbohydrates again. Carbohydrates help the body hold a balanced amount of water. When you consume a high-protein diet at the expense of carbohydrates, your body is unable to hold its water, and you lose mainly water weight. The moment you eat normally again, your body regains the water and retains extra water as a survival reaction. In essence, your body says to itself, "I'd better hold a little extra water in case she does this to me again." Apparently my amazing 10-pound weight loss was merely a temporary water loss.

5. I became even fatter than before my weight loss because the high-protein diet allowed high-fat protein—hamburgers, steaks, pork chops, full-fat cheese, and so on. Since fat is the worst calorie bargain (twice as high in calories as protein or carbohydrate), eating a lot of fat made me gain fat weight *in addition to* water weight.

6. I continued to get fatter, even after I stopped the high-protein diet, because I had deprived my body of needed carbohydrates for two weeks and my body was compelled to overeat quick-fix, simple-sugar, high-fat carbohydrates, such as cookies and doughnuts.

The next diet I tried was a liquid diet in which there is one solid meal a day. I remember drinking my shakes for breakfast and lunch, and obsessing all day about the pitiful "meal" I would get at night. Looking back, I remember it was the size of a frozen foods "dinner." After ten days on this diet, I rebelled, stuffing my face one night, all night long, until I could hardly move.

The next day, after eliminating much of the meal, I continued to binge. I did this for at least ten days, and of course ended up fatter than I was to begin with. But it didn't stop there. I refused to go on any diet for about eight months, and I put on at least another 10 pounds.

My body had rebelled against the liquid diet just as it had against the high-protein diet, but for different reasons. Although the liquid diet boasted a balanced amount of carbohydrates, protein, and fat, my body revolted against not getting enough solid, chewable food. Apparently we were created with the urge to chew food, not merely drink liquids, and if we are denied that urge for any length of time, we find a way to make up for it, and then some. Most people know the story of Oprah, who after carrying a wagon load of fat on national television to demonstrate her miraculous liquid-diet weight loss, ended up gaining more than that amount of fat in less than a year after she went off the diet.

I tried a few more fad diets. There was one where I drank water all day long and kept going to the bathroom, and another where the main fare was grapefruit and eggs. I even tried an ice cream diet. Nothing worked.

HOW I DISCOVERED THE SECRET TO DIETING

Then I ran into bodybuilders at a gym and they told me how they eat. Amazingly, they ate a well-balanced high-carbohydrate, low-fat diet. I tried that diet, and in time modified it in keeping with the USDA'S Food Pyramid. This new eating plan didn't feel like a diet at all. I was able to eat plenty and at the same time lose weight—fat weight, not muscle weight.

The diet I discovered and perfected is contained in this book. It works for me, and it will for you. It is not a fad or a trick diet, but a nutritional combination of foods that will keep your body happy and healthy. You can follow this diet for the rest of your life and remain strong and fit, free of excess body fat. What's more, you'll have more energy than you need to enjoy your life—and you'll never feel hungry. That's a promise.

THE PSYCHOLOGICAL ASPECTS OF OVEREATING

Looking back to the time when I couldn't stop eating, I believe it was more than the physical need to eat that drove me to be overweight. There was a psychological reason as well. I was recently married, and I quickly realized that I had made a mistake. But divorce was anathema in my religion, so I suppressed my unhappiness and began to eat. I clearly remember going upstairs after each week's church service (I was married to a minister). He would be downstairs still greeting people and dealing with church matters. I would raid the refrigerator. Embarrassed that my husband would come up and see me eating so much, I would scarf down as much food as I could, as quickly as possible.

When I would cook or bake, I would consume half the cake or cookie batter, along with most of the frosting, before the goods were baked. I ate and ate and ate. I felt empty and unfulfilled. There was a big void in the center of my being, and I was trying to fill it up with food.

So in addition to my normal urge to eat, triggered by a healthy appetite and habits formulated in a Russian family that believed no one should leave the table quickly (you should be too stuffed to move), I had the psychological element of needing food to fill a void.

It was not until I faced the truth about my unhappy marriage that I was able to even begin getting a grip on my food binges.

DOES FOOD CONTROL YOU?

Ask yourself these questions and give honest answers:

1. How much of my need to eat is due to real hunger?
2. How much of my need to eat is due to the way I was brought up?
3. How much of my need to eat is due to a feeling of empti-

ness in my life—unfulfillment, a lack of love, boredom, frustration?

Real hunger is fine. I can take care of that for you with this diet. You'll have plenty of food to eat, plus extra. No problem.

The way you were brought up, that's habit. You can slowly form new habits if you want to do so. If you were brought up to feel stuffed, there are foods to eat when you need to give in to that urge. You'll form new eating habits by being asked to eat often—and being allowed to eat as often as you wish. In the beginning, you'll be afraid to try this new method. You'll fear that if you eat more often, you'll gain weight. But once you dare to do it, and you see yourself losing weight and not going hungry, you'll be hooked on the new habit.

Now let's talk about the third reason for overeating: the feeling of emptiness inside owing to unfulfilled desires, lack of love, anger, boredom, or frustration. In order to deal with this void, you'll have to take an honest look at your life and admit to yourself what is bothering you. The good news is, just admitting the problem will free you. You'll begin to stop filling that emptiness with food. The next step, of course, is to take action to make your life better, but even just admitting the problem and making plans will enable you to begin changing your eating habits.

If you are not happy with your life and you want to acknowledge what's wrong, answer this question: *Exactly what goes through my mind just before I start putting food in my mouth to binge?*

Your answer may be, "I think I hate my life. I'm trapped in this house with these kids. All I do is work. I never have fun. I deserve some pleasure. I'm going to enjoy this food, damn it." Or your answer may be, "I hate my husband. He never compliments me. He's always criticizing me. No matter what I do, I can never please him, anyway. I might as well eat and enjoy my life."

Your answer may be, "I'm scared I won't pass this difficult course I'm taking. Every time I think of opening up that text, it drives me to eat. I have a hard life. I deserve this food. At least for a moment I can have some pleasure." Or, "There's no use. I'm getting older anyway. Who am I kidding? I can never have the body I dreamed of. It's so sad to get older. It feels as if I'm invisible. Nobody loves me. The hell with it. I might as well eat."

You might say, "I work two jobs and still I can't make ends meet. I have no social life. My date is with the TV. I never get any pleasure. I don't care what I look like—I'm going to give myself something to enjoy. Food is my only pleasure. I can't take that away from myself, for I'll die."

Now, ask yourself if there's anything you can do to at least partially remedy the situation so that you don't feel as frustrated, bored, empty, or angry—and as compelled to eat. Let's take a look at each of the possible answers, then you will see how to apply this kind of thinking to your own situation.

"I hate my life. I'm trapped in this house with these kids. All I do is work. I never have fun. I deserve some pleasure. I'm going to enjoy this food, damn it." Think of what you used to love doing—before you were trapped with the kids. Was it dancing? Arrange for a babysitter and take one dance lesson a week or attend a low-cost or free community dance lesson. Local high schools have jazz, Latin, ballroom, and other types of dancing. If you prefer private or semiprivate lessons and can afford it, look in your Yellow Pages under "Dance" and begin calling around.

Another idea is to forget what you liked to do in the past and think honestly, "What am I really curious about—what would I love to do *now*?" Then order the catalogs for adult education from your local high schools and colleges and enroll in a course of your choosing. It could be anything from *tai chi* to Latin, Chinese cooking to introductory philosophy, or creative writing to French for beginners. You may want to resume an old sport or activity, such as soccer, tennis, or karate, or start a new one, such as yoga, racewalking, or swimming. Add excitement and the feeling of fulfillment to your life. Without realizing it, you will have begun to reward yourself on a daily basis, just for being alive. You will have begun to celebrate your life, your energy, your potential. Gradually, you'll find that food is no longer your only focus.

What if your answer was something like, "I hate my husband. He never compliments me. He's always criticizing me. No matter what I do, I can never please him, anyway. I might as well eat and enjoy my life." You have three choices: (1) insist that your husband go with you to a marriage counselor; (2) go to a psychologist to sort out your feelings; (3) admit to yourself that you made a mistake and begin taking steps to get out of the marriage. We all make mistakes. But we don't have to compound our mistakes by forcing ourselves to live the rest of our lives in misery. I believe that, in fact, life is a test of how we deal with the mistakes we have made! *True* courage is to dare to take action once we realize we have made a big mistake, especially when that action will be difficult and uncomfortable. Free yourself from the burden of an unhappy marriage or relationship, and you will have one less reason to fill that void with food. My book *Get Rid of Him* deals with this issue and can also be read by men in the reverse (see the Bibliography).

Suppose your answer was something like, "I'm scared I won't pass this difficult course I'm taking. Every time I think of opening up that text, it drives me to eat. I have a hard life. I deserve this food. I want to forget my troubles in this food. At least for a moment I can have some pleasure." This one is easier to solve than the first two. First, don't try to approach the text when you are hungry. Eat first. Next, use preconditioning to head off the eating binge. Think ahead. Imagine yourself thinking of opening the book and having the urge to eat instead. Then imagine yourself thinking, "Oh, that's just the frustration urge. Eating won't help and the text has no power to harm me. I'll sit down with the book open for an hour, whether or not I understand what I'm reading. After that, I'll reward myself with an allowed snack. I'll feel good about myself. I'll even make a cup of tea for myself and relax while I read." Then picture yourself opening the book and enjoying an hour or more of reading, and then going for your snack.

Think of feeling good about yourself as you eat your snack, feeling proud that you have accomplished something. Now the next time you're tempted to binge when you think of the text, you'll find your mind going along the preconditioned track. Use preconditioning for other eating situations, too.

♥ What if your answer was something like, "There's no use. I'm getting older anyway. Who am I kidding? I can never have the body I dreamed of. It's so sad to get older. It feels as if I'm invisible. Nobody loves me. Who cares? I might as well eat." Look at me. I'm 53 years old! I have never had a great body even when I was not overweight, and it looked worse as I gained weight. I have bad genetics, yet if I was able to lose weight and reshape my body when I was over 40, you can do it too, and have a better body than you had in your prime. This is a promise. Follow this eating plan, but most important, pick a workout from Chapter 10 and do it. In six months to a year, you will be telling everyone how to get in shape—that's how excited you'll be. Don't be discouraged by your age.

Your answer may be something like, "I work two jobs and still I can't make ends meet. I have no social life. My date is with the TV. I never get any pleasure. I don't care what I look like—I'm going to give myself something to enjoy. Food is my only pleasure. I can't take that away from myself, for I'll die." No matter how busy your schedule, you must arrange an appointment with yourself. Even if it means you have to wait three months for a three-day weekend vacation. You can plan an island escape (there are some real bargains if you book ahead), or you may want to go to Las Vegas. Airlines and hotels have low prices, assuming you are going to gamble. You don't have to gamble, but you can take advantage of the low prices. Another idea is to go to a local health spa, even one in your own town, and spend two or three days getting all kinds of treatments—massages, facials, oil and mineral baths, and so on.

You might not have a day or two to spend, but just a few hours. Make a date with yourself to go some place you enjoy—a museum, botanical garden, zoo, pet shop, flea market. Call a friend and meet for a drink or dinner. If you're single, call an old flame for a reunion. Whatever it is you have the urge to do, indulge yourself. You deserve some pleasure and you can have it.

If you think about it, you may be behaving like a harsh military commander toward yourself, refusing to give yourself even a crumb of enjoyment. What crime did you commit that you treat yourself this way? Small wonder you want to grab a few moments of pleasure by eating extra food. Coax yourself into lightening up. Please, if you don't give yourself a break, who will?

THINK OF YOUR DIET AS: "I'M AN ATHLETE IN TRAINING"— NOT, "I'M BEING DEPRIVED"

One of the biggest problems with dieting is the way we think about it: we feel as if we are being punished. Before we even start the diet, already we are thinking in terms of deprivation. We imagine having constant hunger pangs and picture ourselves eating grass or the equivalent. We resent, way ahead of time, that we will have to give up our goodies, such as greasy hamburgers, doughnuts, cheese, and so on.

But you don't have to think that way. Instead, you can think of your diet as an "I'm in training" food plan. "I'm eating for my muscles." What muscles? The muscles you will make even if you follow the quickest of my workout plans in Chapter 10. But even if you don't choose to work out, think of this diet as being in training for your life—the most important sport of all.

And, anyway, you won't feel deprived for very long. After the initial detoxification, you will no longer constantly crave the fatty, sugary foods you used to eat, because your body will be happier with a nutritionally balanced diet. It will be your mind that from time to time rebels, and later I'll tell you how to deal with this problem. Most important, instead of resenting your diet, you'll soon feel that your new way of eating is a privilege, not a punishment.

It's all about using discipline with a goal in mind, and this kind of discipline can make you feel good about yourself and your life. Think back. Wasn't there a time in your life when you trained for something? Even though you had to pay a price for that training, you enjoyed the discipline and felt good about yourself doing it. Maybe you were on the track team in school, where you had to run a certain distance every day and eat certain foods to ensure your energy levels. Perhaps your discipline had nothing to do with sports. You may have been in a choral group, where you had to practice a lot and take care of your voice. Maybe you were in a dance group at school or in plays. In either case, you had to use discipline—to take care of yourself, to put in time to practice—and you did it because you knew you were in training for something special.

Athletes train all the time. Boxers, football players, dancers, marathon runners all discipline themselves and eat a certain way because they are "in training." Adapt an "I'm in training" attitude. When you find yourself reaching for those foods that made you fat in the first place, instead of feeling depressed and punished, you'll think, "No. I can't have that. I'm in training." And you'll smile and think of yourself as special and disciplined. You'll actually love yourself in these moments.

USE VISUALIZATION AND PRECONDITIONING

Other techniques to help you keep on your diet include visualization. Continually visualize your body evolving into its perfect form. Start by sitting in a quiet place. See your naked body in the mirror the way it looks now. Then imagine yourself looking at your naked body one month later. Notice that your body has gotten smaller, that there is noticeably less fat. Imagine yourself feeling proud and happy, even excited. "Tell" your body to evolve into that reduced form.

Now picture yourself again looking in the mirror at your nude body another month later. See yourself being surprised to notice that your body seems to be shrinking—getting smaller, the fat disappearing. Imagine yourself experiencing a feeling of joy and power. "I can do this. It works. I'm proud of myself." "Tell" your body to continue to evolve into that reduced form.

Now picture yourself a third month later, again looking in the mirror at your naked body and seeing yet more reduction in size and fat. Imagine yourself feeling even more powerful and in control. Imagine a feeling of solidity rising from the center of your being. "Tell" your body to continue losing weight and feeling better.

Picture yourself six months later (or a year if you think you need more time). Imagine your body at your ideal weight. Imagine yourself feeling as if you have achieved a wonderful thing. Imagine yourself remaining in control of your eating for life. "Tell" your body to reach its goal in a year's time (or three months, or six months, whichever is realistic for you). Mark your goal date on the calendar. Every month, look at your naked body in the mirror and see your progress. Continue to "tell" your body to move toward its goal. In one year, mark on the calendar your new weight. But much more important, take a photograph of yourself in a bathing suit or underwear before you start your diet, and one on your goal date.

The next technique that helps you keep to your diet is preconditioning. You can precondition yourself to resist eating the wrong foods. Imagine yourself following the eating plan in this book for a few days, and then picture yourself looking in the refrigerator at the ice cream container (your husband, who is not on the diet, insists upon having his "goodies" around). Envision yourself at the freezer door with the spoon in your hand, opening the container, digging in, scooping up a spoon, ready to lift it to your mouth. With that action, imagine a feeling of nausea waving over you. Imagine yourself feeling too sick to eat the ice cream.

Now imagine yourself cutting up red peppers, tomatoes, and cucumbers and sprinkling them with vinegar and spices. Picture yourself eating until you're full and feeling great about yourself afterwards for having eaten the right foods.

To add to your preconditioning power, go back to the ice

cream. Picture yourself again ready to raise the spoon of ice cream to your mouth, and imagine with that action a feeling of anger and the thought arising, "No. I won't do it. This ice cream is not worth my depression and feeling fat all the time." Then imagine yourself thinking, "I can have ice cream once a week when I reach my goal—without guilt. It's worth the wait. I can wait. I can make a snack that will be filling right now. At least I don't have to go hungry." And with that, picture yourself putting the ice cream back or throwing the spoon with the ice cream into the sink and closing the freezer, and making yourself a healthful snack.

List the foods you will be most tempted by and the situations in which you are likely to run into these foods. Go through this process for each food and situation, preconditioning yourself so that when the time comes, you will be one step ahead of yourself.

BE ONE STEP AHEAD OF YOURSELF

Instead of making it hard on yourself, make it easy! Once you become familiar with the food plan in this book, keep a supply of allowed foods on hand at all times. Carry Baggies of carrot, red pepper, and cucumber strips, whole wheat bread slices, fruit, and so on. Keep a loaf of whole wheat bread and cans of tuna in water in your desk drawer at work, along with some bottled water. These items don't have to be refrigerated, and you'll have no excuse to accept the offer of chocolate candy from your deskmate. Work with, rather than against, yourself.

Do the same thing at home. If you know you're tempted to snack the moment you get home from work or after a long day outside with the children, have a bowl of precut snacks ready in the refrigerator. This way you won't go straight for the jar of peanut butter. I'll give you lots of easy snack ideas in Chapters 3 to 9.

Instead of setting yourself up for failure, create an environment that will nudge you toward success!

REVERSE ANY NEGATIVE SELF-TALK

Why are we so mean to ourselves? We tell ourselves things like, "You have no willpower," "You're hopeless," "Who are you kidding? You'll always be a fat slob." What if someone actually said these things to you? You wouldn't take it, would you? But you say these things to yourself—in your own mind or even out loud when no one is around. Sometimes you even say negative things about yourself to others.

Well, you can stop such negative self-talk by using five simple steps. The next time you catch yourself saying something bad about yourself, whether it's in your own mind, out loud to yourself, or to others, do the following:

1. Write down the negative statement about yourself on paper.

2. Take a pen and draw a line through the statement, crossing it out as wrong the way your English teacher would if you made a mistake in your composition.

3. Look at the crossed-out statement and say out loud, "No." Think in your mind, "This is not true. This is a lie I tell myself."

4. Between the crossed-out lines, write a new, positive statement about yourself. Base it upon past experience in areas when you demonstrated excellent behavior or, by faith, simply project future positive behavior.

5. Think about the new statement and remember times when you demonstrated that behavior, and/or picture yourself behaving that way in the future.

Let's see how this works by way of example. You just ate a forbidden food and you said in your mind, "I have no willpower." Write it down: "I have no willpower." Now cross it out and at the same time, think about the statement and say out loud, "No. It's not true. This is a lie I've told myself." Then write down, "I have great willpower when I want to use it. I get up at 6:00 every morning and go to work in bad weather, when

I'm tired, even when I feel sick." Realize that you have excellent willpower, and that you can use that willpower to change your eating habits, just as you use that willpower in other areas. Picture yourself willfully eating the foods that are allowed on the eating plan and refusing to give in to urges to eat foods that will take you off course.

Whenever you catch yourself thinking or verbalizing defeatist thoughts about yourself, take the time to use this method. In time, you'll find that your unconscious message to yourself is uplifting rather than draining. You'll have more energy to achieve your goals.

FEAR OF SUCCESS

You may have heard of the psychological phenomenon "fear of success." Psychologists have discovered that some people, in spite of intelligence, talent, drive, and creativity, sometimes set themselves up for failure by putting obstacles in their way to make sure that they won't succeed. Such people often do not realize that the reason for their failure is not "the world," but themselves. Why do they do this?

Psychologists agree that many people do this because, deep down inside, they feel that if they did succeed, more would be expected of them, and they wonder whether they could live up to those expectations. So every time they are about to make a move toward career advancement, financial success, or some such achievement they unconsciously set themselves up for failure. They may come late for an important business meeting that would have meant a promotion, get into an argument at work with people who have the power to determine their future, disregard intelligent advice regarding a foolish investment, and so on. There are literally thousands of ways our unconscious can sabotage our efforts if we believe it must be so to protect ourselves.

Well, the same phenomenon can be at work when it comes to weight loss. Some people are afraid that if they lose weight, more will be expected of them. They imagine that their whole lives will change. They envision people giving them more attention, and they wonder if they can cope with this scrutiny. They realize that if they lose weight, new opportunities for romance, career advancement, a social life—who knows what else—may open up, and this scares them to death.

When such people begin a diet, they do fine. But after a few weeks or months—whenever the fear of success begins to kick in—their unconscious takes over and impels them to sabotage their efforts. Suddenly they break their diets and eventually they overeat until they regain all the lost weight and are once again safely hidden by the comforting known—the cover of fat.

⸙ Yes, losing weight will cause a change in your life. And change, for most people, is in and of itself sometimes scary. When you lose weight, you may well get more attention from the opposite sex. You may feel that you're not ready for that attention, or you may wonder if you'll be able to live up to that attention. If you're in a relationship or marriage, you may sense that your spouse secretly likes you to be fat. On some level, you may intuit that if you lose weight, your mate will become insecure and threatened, and cause trouble.

You may have friends and relatives who have been encouraging you to lose weight, but on some level you wonder how your relationship with them might change if you did lose that weight. Would they be happy for you—or in some ways, would they become competitive with you instead of the sympathetic supporters they are now? These thoughts can scare you into backtracking to the safety of overweight.

Then there are anxieties regarding your career. If you lose weight, you'll not only look healthier and more appealing to the eye, but you'll have more energy and a more positive approach to situations. When this is noticed, more opportunities will come your way—you may be offered new challenges. Will you be able to live up to them? If you do take on the challenge and succeed, will your life change still more? Are you ready for major changes in your life? You think, "Maybe it's better to stay in the cocoon of the known—to remain enveloped in the womb of this soft pillow of fat. This way, not much will be expected of me."

What can you do if you think this may be your problem? For starters, you can catch yourself in the act of sabotaging your diet. The next time you cheat on your diet, ask yourself exactly what is going through your mind. If it's a thought like, "I don't want to be thin anyway. Who needs all that attention? It's shallow people who look at the exterior," chances are you have this problem.

What can you do about it? Argue back. Say, "No. It has nothing to do with shallow people. It has to do with my natural fear of change and challenges. I'll cross that bridge when I come to it. I'm not going to chicken out this time. Life is too short to waste it on worrying about my weight. I want to get this out of the way now—once and for all."

If you find that you can't talk yourself out of it, and no matter what you do you keep sabotaging your diet for fear of success, you may want to see a psychologist, who can help you get at the root of your problem. See my books *Look In, Look Up, Look Out! Be the Person You Were Meant to Be* and *Get Rid of Him*, listed in the Bibliography, for suggestions on how to find the right psychologist.

FEAR OF DEALING WITH THE REAL ISSUES OF LIFE

A closely related psychological phenomenon to the fear of success is the fear of facing life. Often, people sabotage their efforts to lose weight because they don't want to face the real issues. Such people spend most of their psychological energy obsessing about their weight problem. When they think of losing weight, deep down inside, they realize that when they no longer have "the problem," when their bodies are at the right weight, they will be forced to deal with the issues at hand: what to do about their careers, their relationships, their goals in life, and so on. Because such people are afraid to confront these issues, they make sure they always have a bigger, more obvious problem to deal with—the mountain of fat.

OVEREXPECTATIONS FROM WEIGHT LOSS

Now let's talk about the opposite problem. Suppose you don't have a fear of success or a fear of dealing with the real issues. Suppose you really *want* to lose weight and have in fact succeeded on other diets. But for some mysterious reason, after a time, you always gain it back. If this is you, you may be suffering from unrealistic expectations about weight loss. Here's how it works.

People who are fat for a number of years often tell themselves, "If only I could lose this weight, I would meet someone, I would get a better job, I wouldn't have to put up with. . . ." But when they lose the weight, they don't immediately meet the person of their dreams, they don't get an instant promotion, and in fact many of their problems are still the same.

To deal with this, think ahead. Realize that losing weight will improve your life on many levels, but it is not a cure-all. You will feel and look better, and in general people will react more positively toward you. You will have more energy and will have a more positive approach to life. However, there will still be people who reject you. You'll still have struggles in your career, and there will always be the normal problems of daily life.

The bottom line is, don't expect too much from weight loss. It's a great beginning, but it's *just* a beginning. It will free you to focus attention on the real challenges of life, but it will not ensure that you will "live happily ever after." If that were true, every thin person would be walking around with a blissful smile.

NO DIETING UNTIL YOU DO THE MENTAL PREPARATION

Before you start your diet, take time to do some psychological preparation. Make your unconscious ready for dieting.

1. Read the text in Chapters 3 through 10 of this book and skim through the recipes. Underline sentences and paragraphs that strike you. Make comments and notes in the margin. Make it yours.

2. After reading Chapter 10, decide which exercise plan you will follow. You may want to start the exercise plan the same week you start the diet. Or start the diet first, and exactly one week later (no longer than that), start the exercise plan.

3. Mark your start date on the calendar. Most people feel more comfortable starting diets and exercise plans on the weekend or on a Monday. You decide what's best for you.

4. Review the recipes and meal plans (Chapters 5 to 9) and decide which plan you will follow the first week. To make it simple, follow the meal plans in the order presented. You won't repeat a meal for a whole month!

5. A few days before your start date, do your food shopping based upon the meal plans chosen for your first week.

6. The night before you start your diet, take fifteen minutes of private time to calmly think about the beginning of a new life. Skim through the book, look at your calendar with the date circled, and tell yourself that this is a new beginning. Tell yourself to relax and calmly lose the weight. Remind yourself that getting the weight off is not a police emergency. It didn't come upon you overnight, although it may seem to have done so. (No one gains even 2 pounds a week—104 pounds a year—do they?)

7. Decide how much you expect to lose each month. Don't go by the week because body weight varies from week to week, depending upon water retention and other factors. Frankly, a nice, easy way is to make 5 to 10 pounds a month your goal. You may well lose more, but 5 to 10 pounds a month will ensure that your body is comfortable giving up the weight and it does not rebel and force you to overeat to regain the weight.

SHHH. DON'T TALK ABOUT IT TOO SOON!

When you're about to start a new diet, it's a good idea to keep it to yourself—unless you have a trusted friend who will be supportive. Here's how to tell whether or not you should let your friend in on your new plan. Imagine yourself starting the diet and keeping it for a few days, and then breaking it and eating all the wrong foods. Picture your friend calling and asking, "How are you doing on the diet?" How would you feel? Would you be too ashamed to tell her? If so, don't tell this person about your diet. On the other hand, if you could expect a supportive, encouraging remark, such as, "Don't worry. Just get up and start again. We all stumble sometimes. It's not the short run, but the long run that counts," then you can tell this friend.

Don't tell too many people until you've been on the diet for two to three weeks. It's hard enough to get used to a new way of eating. Why involve others who may plant seeds of doubt or may not wish you well? In addition, the more people you tell, the more psychological pressure you may feel to measure up. You may begin to picture the people you told watching you, mocking you if you go off the diet and look as fat as ever the next time you see them. All of this may become too much for you, and you may say to yourself, "The hell with it. I don't need this," and you may throw the diet out the window.

Better to wait until new eating habits have had a chance to take root. You'll know when to start telling people. Probably it will be once they start noticing your weight loss. For lots of other methods to keep yourself on this weight-loss plan, see *Look In, Look Up, Look Out!* (listed in the Bibliography).

SOMETHING TO LOOK FORWARD TO

Here's some good news. Once you reach your weight goal, you'll have a break. You'll be able to choose between two plans of maintaining your weight loss. Plan A will allow you to eat a little something previously forbidden once a day. Plan B will allow you to save up your "forbidden" allotment and eat it in more abundance once a week. Much more about this later, but for now, suffice it to say that no matter what your dream "naughty" food is, you can have it at some point. You don't have to permanently kiss it good-bye (unless your doctor advises against it for medical reasons. This applies to everyone, but especially to those people with heart conditions). And because you will at some point be able to have your "goodies," you won't be caught up in obsessing about that food, and won't feel resentful and deprived. These foods will become a normal, unintimidating part of your life. *Vedral's Believe It or Not!*

THE PSYCHOLOGY OF UNLIMITED HEALTHFUL FOODS

What about telling people that, when they feel they must, it's okay to eat until stuffed? This is part of the diet too, although you are allowed to eat only certain low-fat complex carbohydrates. With these foods, you can stuff yourself all day long and still lose weight. But isn't this teaching people to not have discipline and to misuse food?

No, the opposite is true. By satisfying the psychological urge to put food in their mouths when they feel they must fill their stomachs, people avoid letting food become an obsession. At least dieters know that they do not have to go hungry.

As discussed before, your hunger may not be based upon physical need but on a psychological one: the need to fill a void in your life. But that need is just as real as if it were physical. And what are you to do while working on those psychological problems? Once you have used up your food allotment for the day, should you bite the bullet and eat nothing until the next day? No, that would be asking too much. Instead, I give you foods that you can eat in unlimited quantities, day or night—red or green peppers, cucumbers, broccoli, cauliflower, and so on. This way you never have to feel deprived. It's better than nothing, trust me, and it's good for your health to boot.

When I was on various food-allotment diets, I would use up my allotment for the day, even though it was only 6 o'clock in the evening. Not only would I feel dread, I would experience a sense of fear. Knowing that I could not eat until the next day made me feel insecure and afraid. On those days I would try to go to bed early so that my temptation time would be limited. And worse, on the days when I gave in and ate something, I would feel like a failure and binge the entire next day.

So I offer you food that you can eat anytime, anywhere, and in any amount. I know that if I didn't have that option I would give up any idea of dieting and just eat what I wanted and be fat. Because even though I have dealt with my psychological reasons for overeating, I'm still human, and there are some days when psychological needs take over and I just want to eat!

I notice that I feel this way when I'm frustrated, bored, or lonely. I could talk to myself and find out the root cause, but I don't feel like analyzing myself to death. I just want to eat. On those occasions, I thank God I can eat food that will not break my diet—that I can still lose weight, even though my stomach is stuffed. I'll show you exactly how to do this in Chapters 5 to 9.

BEFORE AND AFTER—THIS COULD BE YOU

Myself and the following people are only a few of the thousands of examples of those who have lost weight and kept it off by following the reasonable, realistic, nonpunishing eating plan presented in this book. We all work out in addition to following the eating plan, but none of us works out for hours a day. We follow a reasonable exercise plan—anywhere from twenty to forty minutes a day. And the medical community is in full agreement with that idea—a reasonable exercise plan is important if you want to keep the weight off!

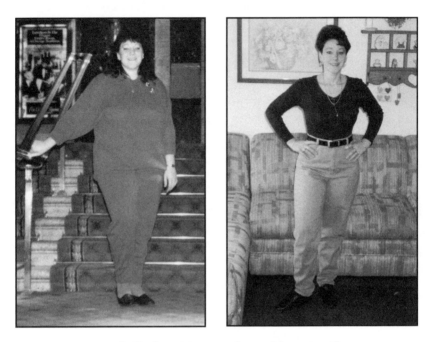

Michelle lost 90 pounds and kept it off.
From size 22–24 to size 10–12.

Michelle Lost 90 Pounds,
From Size 22–24 to Size 10–12 in Fourteen Months

Michelle was very overweight—nearly a hundred pounds. By following the eating plan in this book and doing a combination of my workouts (*Bottoms Up!* and *Definition*), she not only lost the weight but got tight and toned.

Michelle is 28. She has a three-year-old son, and she also works as a data processor, so she is very busy and often uses the quick meals for herself, reserving her cooking time for her family.

Michelle's husband is both proud and relieved. He feels that now Michelle is not burdened by thinking of her weight all the time, and he has been overheard telling people that Joyce Vedral's program works. The best part of the eating plan, Michelle says, is "I eat all the time—within reason. I don't eat Twinkies. If I want a snack I treat myself to a fat-free ice cream or a big bowl of hard pretzels, or a bowl of hot-air popcorn with some Butter Buds. I snack every night. I eat three snacks a day plus my three meals. I used to be very self-conscious of eating at restaurants before. People would look at me and think, 'She really needs to get that salad.' But now I know it's not the salad I need. I can have a big fat potato or a big plate of spaghetti—a salad goes along with that. I never have to worry, 'I can't have any more to eat today.'" As Michelle does, if you've used up your food allotment, there are always the free unlimited complex carbohydrates.

Michelle notes, "You have to think ahead. If I know I'm not going to be able to stop to eat, I carry a lunch—a Baggy with Joyce's muffins, carrot sticks, a juicy orange, cans of tuna packed in water. I think the major thing to remember is take your own salad dressing to the restaurant. In the restaurant you learn to tell them 'I'll have it on the side.' If people look at me, I don't care. When I'm as big as the couch, then that's my problem! The bottom line is, now I can live my life and forget about food—food is no longer an issue."

Kathy Lost 62 Pounds, From Size 16 to Size 4 in Seven Months

Kathy is the mother of two children aged 11 and 8. She used to wear a hefty size 16 jeans, and in her own words, "they fit more like panty hose than jeans." Now she wears a size 4 and there's room in them to move. What's more, Kathy has just completed modeling school and is looking toward a new career. In her own words, "I feel as if I've been transformed from an 'ugly duckling' into a beautiful swan. I've been freed to enjoy and appreciate life in ways I never knew possible. The

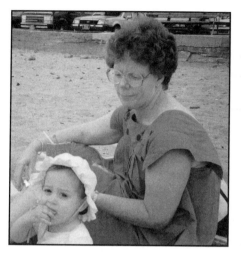

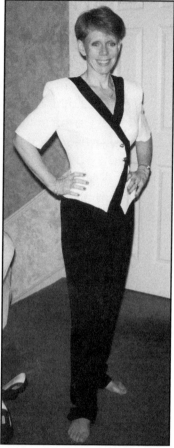

Kathy lost 62 pounds after seven months and kept it off. From size 16 to size 4.

direct result of enhancing my 'exterior' beauty has been to enhance my inner beauty."

Kathy did the workout in *Bottoms Up!* and *The Fat-Burning Workout* along with the eating plan in this book. "In the beginning I cheated a little, but I followed the basic plan. What I mean is, I would eat, say, a few extra no-fat dairies in place of the limited complex carbohydrates—but I would have more than I should. Of course, I still lost weight because I was so fat to begin with. But looking at the basic guidelines of the food groups is what helped me so much. Even if I didn't get it exactly right in the beginning, I still lost so much weight, because my body was finally getting a much better food balance. Now, over two years later, I'm keeping the weight off and it's not a problem. The funny thing is, I can't eat the way I used to even if I tried. The other day I tasted a spoonful of peanut butter and it made me sick. Before, I used to eat it by the jar. Another example—I tried to eat chicken Parmesan at a restaurant and the cheese made me sick. Your body gets addicted to good food. I don't even like the taste of full-fat ice cream or milk anymore."

The best part of this diet? "Well, let's just say the other day I almost didn't buy a pair of sexy tight leggings—my old thinking was trying to dominate. I thought I'd be self-conscious. Then I said, 'Hey, why not?' My hips used to be 44 inches; now they're 35. I bought them, and sure enough the first day I wore them I noticed that some heads were turning—good-looking men were noticing. And I'm in my forties, feeling younger and sexier than ever."

Dana Lost 34 Pounds, From Size 13 After Pregnancy Weight to Size 4 in Fourteen Weeks

Dana is a registered nurse working in labor and delivery. When Dana became pregnant, she had to stay in bed because of pregnancy complications, so she gained more weight than she had hoped. She was 164 pounds just before she gave birth. After the baby she lost only 10 pounds, leaving her at 154 pounds—and a hefty size 13. So Dana decided to follow the eating plan in this book (she also did my *Definition* workout). In fourteen weeks, she weighed in at 120 pounds and was the size 4 of her dreams. "I have never been a size 4 in my life. The smallest I've ever been was a 10." But what makes Dana happiest of all is not so much her weight loss but the career that has opened up for her. Like Kathy, she is now pursuing the modeling that she had put off for years because she was unable to lose weight. "I'm loving every minute of it," says Dana, "and I've been getting plenty of modeling jobs, too."

She explains, "This food plan taught me the basic principles of healthful weight-loss eating. You have no idea how ill-

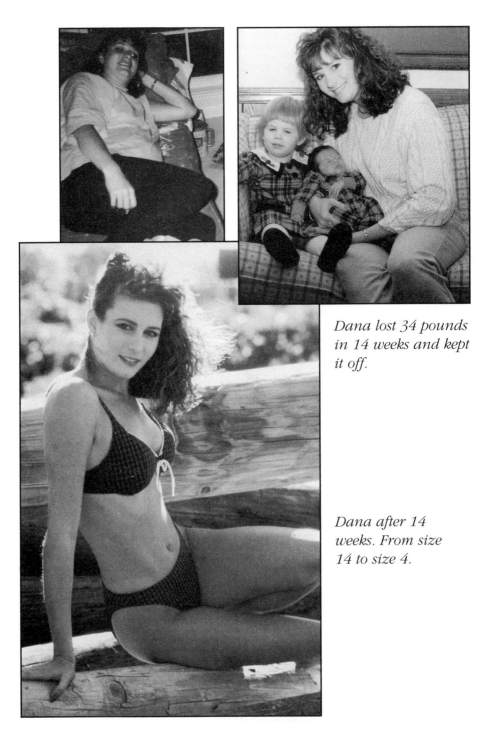

Dana lost 34 pounds in 14 weeks and kept it off.

Dana after 14 weeks. From size 14 to size 4.

informed I was before. Do you believe that before this diet I used to consume a few glasses of juice with each meal—orange juice, apple juice. Then I read Joyce's advice on not drinking so much juice, but that it's a better idea to eat the fruit instead, because of the bulk and fiber. I gave up the many glasses of juice and followed the plan. Right there I started to lose weight. I also used to eat a lot of cheese. I didn't feel full—I just ate a few slices at a time, a few times a day. All that fat added up and I guess that's why I couldn't lose weight. I didn't think I was eating that much because I also ate healthy—vegetables— but they were cooked with butter. After reading Joyce's plan, I realized that the butter had to go, too.

"Funny, before I wasn't eating that much food, so I didn't know why I was so fat. Now I know why I was fat. And the amazing part is, I now eat much more food, I feel more satisfied, and I am three sizes smaller than I was at my best—and five sizes smaller than when I was at my worst! The best part of it all is, I don't ever feel hungry. I'm a nurse and I know about good nutrition, and let me tell you, this plan is good nutrition. My body tells me so every day."

Wes Lost 23 Pounds, From Size 38 Pants to Size 33 in Nine Months

Wes used to weigh 187 pounds. After following the eating plan in this book and doing the workout found in *Top Shape* and *Gut Busters*, he's now 165 pounds. What's more, Wes's blood pressure and cholesterol, which were both in the danger zone, are now in the perfect zone. Even his doctor is amazed.

"Before I started this eating plan I used to eat tons of chips and cookies and so many hamburgers they used to call me 'Wimpy.' I not only looked bloated and heavy, but I felt that way—at 52 I felt like an old man. Now I feel like a man half my age and I'm full of energy. I look at other people my age who are overweight and out of shape the way I used to be, and

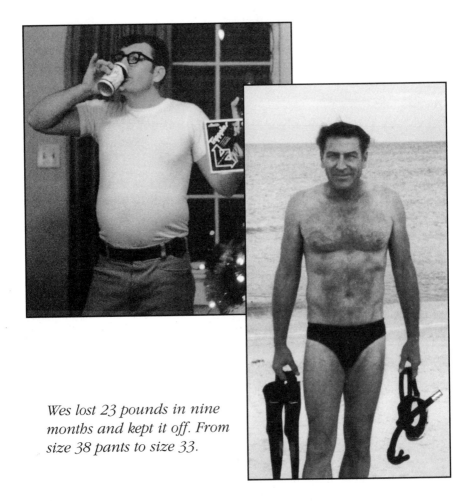

Wes lost 23 pounds in nine months and kept it off. From size 38 pants to size 33.

I feel so sorry for them, knowing that I have the answer for them, but like me, they have to find it for themselves.

"I learned not only to follow the food plan but to read labels. Now I look at the labels in the supermarket and I see 'too much fat' or 'too much sodium.' I also notice the portions. They give you such small ones that you usually have to triple them—you know that one portion is never going to be enough to fill you up. Oh, another thing—I used to eat three heavy meals a day, all fat. Now I eat five or six meals a day—exactly like Joyce says—and I'm more satisfied."

Wes is now engaged to a woman in her late twenties!

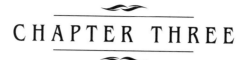

CHAPTER THREE

ALL ABOUT FOOD—AND THE EATING PLAN

Carbohydrates, protein, fat: grams, percentage, saturated, unsaturated, polyunsaturated. Cholesterol: good, bad. Fiber, vitamins, minerals: calcium, sodium—and on and on. What's a person to do? What do you *really* have to know in order to make sure you're getting a balanced diet and still lose weight?

Well, if you take my word for it and just follow the meal plans in Chapter 9, you don't have to know anything. But it's much better if you know *why* you are being asked to eat a certain way. If you know why, at some point in the future you'll be able to eat right on your own—make your own meal plans, so to speak—without sitting down and writing them out.

The goal of this chapter is to provide you with the basic information you need about food, including how to read food labels. But most important, I explain exactly how the eating plan works and why it is a balanced diet that will encourage your body to enjoy healthy foods on a regular basis—foods that will ensure that while you never go hungry, your body will give up its fat storage so that you can once and forever be the healthy weight you want to be.

CALORIES: NEEDED FOR SURVIVAL—AND HOW WE GAIN AND LOSE WEIGHT

Calories come from the food you eat. They are necessary to provide energy so that your body can function. When you eat and digest any food, calories—units of energy—are released to your body. If you eat just the right number of calories, your body uses them up for daily functions such as walking, reading, even breathing. You neither gain nor lose weight. If you don't eat enough calories, your body begins to use up its stored body fat to provide energy and you lose weight. Your body consumes one pound of stored body fat for every 3,500 calories it uses up. If you stop eating completely, eventually your body will consume all its excess fat, and then will start working on its muscle tissue. In time, your body will consume itself and you will die of malnutrition.

But what happens if you eat too many calories? Your body does the reverse. It enlarges itself, gaining weight by storing the excess calories as fat in favorite storage bins such as the stomach, hip, butt, thighs, even on the back, arms, face, and neck—everywhere! How much excess body fat can you store? I recently heard of a woman who weighed a thousand pounds.

But wait a minute. Why am I talking about calories? Isn't it true that the only way you can get fat is by overeating fat? No. You can also gain weight by overeating other foods—carbohydrates and proteins—but it's much easier to gain weight if you overeat fat. Fat calories are more than twice as "fat" as other calories, yet little energy is used up in the digestion of fats. What does this mean?

WHY FAT IS "FATTER" THAN PROTEIN OR CARBOHYDRATES

Fat contains 9 calories per gram, while protein and carbohydrates contain only 4 calories per gram. In other words, you get more than twice as fat by eating fat grams than you do if you eat carbohydrate or protein grams. But there's more to it than that. Very little energy is consumed when the body processes fat. In other words, when you eat fat, almost all of it goes right to energy or storage in the body. Only 3 percent of the fat calories consumed is used up in the digestion process, whereas about 20 percent of protein and carbohydrate calories are used up in the digestion process.

To explain how this works, let's take an example of eating 100 calories of pure fat—butter. Your body uses up 3 percent, or 3 calories, in the digestive process and the remaining 97 percent, or 97 calories, are available for use either as energy or storage in the form of body fat. Now suppose you instead eat 100 calories of carbohydrates—whole wheat bread. Your body uses up 20 percent of those calories in the digestion process and only 80 of those calories are available for use as energy or storage. So from a weight-loss standard, not to mention for health reasons that will be discussed later, it's a good idea to keep your daily fat intake to a minimum. But how much fat will you be allowed?

FAT: YOU WON'T HAVE TO FIGURE PERCENTAGES

After I explain percentages to you—once and for all—I'm not going to talk percentage, I'm going to talk grams. It's much easier to add up your daily fat grams than to figure out the percentage of fat you eat in every food.

It's not just that I want to save you the complicated math. Sometimes a food may have a seemingly high percentage of fat for the total calorie count of the portion, yet it may be well worth your while to have that food. Nutritionists agree that, as a general rule, since you want to keep your total daily fat intake to 20 percent or less, it's not a good idea to consume a food that gets more than 20 percent of its calories from fat. Their reasoning is that if the dieter makes sure that no given food in a day has more than 20 percent fat, he or she cannot go over a total daily consumption of more than 20 percent fat. This is one way of doing it, but in my opinion it is a burdensome way.

My method is more liberating and much more simple. I tell you from the outset that all you have to do is not go over a certain number of fat grams. Women are allowed a maximum of 25 grams of fat a day; men, 30 to 40 grams. If you are a woman and you don't eat more than 25 grams of fat in a day, and you follow the food guidelines in this book, you could never consume more than 20 percent fat. In fact, you'll never go over 15 percent fat. I'll do the math for you later, but for now let me tell you exactly why I would hate my life if I were forbidden to consume any food that had over 20 percent fat.

A typical favorite food of mine that I practically live on are the Classico sauces that I put on pasta or even whole wheat toast. My favorite Classico sauce, Mushrooms and Ripe Olives, has 2 grams of fat per serving and 50 calories a serving. When I figure out the percentage of fat by using division, I discover that this food item has 36 percent fat. If I were forbidden to eat anything with more than 20 percent fat, I wouldn't be able to enjoy my sauce. What do I care that the particular item has a high fat percentage? For two measly grams of fat—only 2 out of an allotment of 25—I can enjoy my life. And I can even have two servings, for 4 grams of fat as long as my diet is balanced and I don't go over my total allotment of 25 grams for the day. And the amazing part is, if I did double the portion, I would have only 4 grams of fat and 100 calories—and think of how I would enjoy that juicy pasta with a whole cup of sauce on it!

Let me give you one more example of how wonderful it is not to worry about percentages of fat. Suppose your day has nearly ended and you've consumed only 19 grams of fat. Your husband is merrily eating oat crackers and you want some, too. You look at the box and note that the crackers have 100 calories for a serving of 22 small crackers, and there are 3 grams of fat per serving. Twenty-seven calories of fat (9 calories per gram) equals 27 percent of the total calorie content. If you had to worry that the food item was over 20 percent fat, you couldn't eat it. But now you can because you say to yourself, "Hey, I still have 1 definite gram of fat left and an additional 5 optional grams. I'll take my fat gram that's coming to me for the minimum of 20 a day, plus 2 optional fat grams and I'm still under my maximum of 25 grams of fat."

Before I go any further, I want to prove to you that on this diet you will never go over your allowed daily percentage of fat. As an example, consider a woman who chooses to consume the lower range of the fat allowance, 20 grams. Since fat has 9 calories a gram, she will consume 180 calories in fat. If she eats 1,800 calories for the day (the other foods will be protein and carbohydrates), she will have consumed only 10 percent of her daily food intake in fat (divide 180 by 1,800 to get the percentage).

But chances are she won't always eat 1,800 calories in a day. She may consume only 1,200 calories on a given day. Then her daily fat intake will be 15 percent of her total intake—still well under the recommended maximum of 20 percent. On another day she may again consume 1,800 calories, but this time she may take advantage of her maximum fat allowance—25. Let's see what happens then. Twenty-five grams of fat contain 225 calories. Once you do the math, you see that she's consumed only 12 percent of her total calorie intake in fat.

If this is so, how then would a person ever go as high as the 15 percent maximum, which, as mentioned above, is really very low? Well, suppose you consume 1,500 calories for the day and eat the maximum amount of fat grams—25, or 225 calories. Your total fat percentage intake for the day would be 15 percent. By way of review, I did the math by dividing the total fat grams for the day by the total calories for the day. And, yes, I used a calculator and even so, I got a headache.

Do you see how neat my calculation-free system is? No matter what you do, if you follow the food guidelines you will never go above 15 percent fat for the day. But doesn't that depend upon how many calories you consume? Yes, but you will rarely go above 1,800 calories because the foods allowed on this diet are rather low in calories, even though they are filling. And I want to remind you that if you follow the meal plans in Chapters 5 to 9, you won't have to count anything—not even fat grams. It's all done for you. This information is for the future—when you make up your own meal plans.

Where will you get your 20 to 25 grams of fat a day? There is no special list of "fat foods" to eat to satisfy your daily allotment. Most of your fat grams will automatically come from protein, but as you will note by reading food labels, there's fat in most foods, and those fat grams add up quickly!

Why We Need Some Fat in Our Diet

We must consume a certain amount of fat on a daily basis in order to be healthy. If there is a significant fat deficit in the body, we cannot absorb and make use of calcium or vitamins A, D, E, or K. If we completely deprive our bodies of fat, our internal organs will have no cushioning. It is fat that composes the major part of the cell membrane and sex hormones.

How much fat is needed for healthy bodily functions? Ten percent of total daily consumption is the bare minimum and 15 percent is a comfortable minimum. You will notice that sometimes the daily meal plans add up to less than 20 grams of fat. This is no problem because it is never less than the 10 percent requirement. The U.S. government had put out a 30 percent recommendation, but most doctors disagree with this for health reasons. For purposes of losing weight, a 30 percent fat intake is way too much. Imagine what happens to the average American whose diet consists of 45 percent fat!

"Good Fat" Versus Bad Fat

When it comes to losing weight, there's no such thing as "good fat." It is not uncommon to have a waiter in a restaurant swear up and down to me that the fish is broiled with no fat. When I get the fish and it's obviously been well oiled, and I challenge him, he reverently and with great assurance says, "Oh, but that's olive oil—it's good fat." Does he mean it won't make me fat? Fat chance!

You won't have to worry about good or bad fat. For our purposes, generally speaking, all fat is bad. Except, of course, your allotment, which will usually come from your daily protein requirement, and here you'll have some choices—more about that later. But there are rare occasions when I do ask you to cook with a teaspoon of canola or olive oil. I do this only when you would otherwise fall below your daily minimum fat gram allowance. However, if you occasionally fall below that minimum, no harm will be done; if it really bothers you, leave out the canola oil.

I also allow you to occasionally have the 1 percent fat cheese, cream cheese, cottage cheese, or milk. I allow this only on days when otherwise your fat allowance would fall too low.

Saturated, Monounsaturated, Polyunsaturated, and "Trans" Fats

Although all fats will make you equally fat, as far as your health goes, the worst type of fat is saturated fat, found in animal products, such as red meat, egg yolks, and full-fat dairy products, and tropical oils, such as palm oil, coconut oil, and cocoa butter. These fats all become solid or semisolid at room temperature. Can you imagine what they do in your arteries if consumed in any significant amount? You got it. They clog your arteries. In addition, they tend to raise your "bad" (low-density lipoprotein, LDL) cholesterol level (more about cholesterol later).

The unsaturated fats fall into two groups: monounsaturated and polyunsaturated. Let's talk about the "mono's" first. This fat is found in avocado and also olive, canola, peanut, and almond oil. It does not become solid at room temperature and does not clog your arteries. When used to replace saturated fats, it tends to increase good cholesterol (high-density lipoprotein, HDL) and lower bad cholesterol (LDL levels). But remember, these fats will make you just as fat as other fats.

Now let's talk about polyunsaturated fats—corn, safflower, sesame, soybean, sunflower, and walnut oil as well as the fats in certain fish, such as herring, oysters, mackerel, salmon, sardines, and whitefish. (These are high-fat fish and are not recommended while you're trying to lose weight. Except for salmon and swordfish, valued for their Omega 3 fatty acids, they are not included in this meal plan. Omega 3 is a food element said to be good for the heart, but you'll get plenty of Omega 3 if you eat canned tuna in water, especially if you choose white meat over light, and in the occasional salmon and swordfish in the meal plans.)

Up until recently, the polyunsaturated fats have also been touted as healthy because they tend to lower bad (LDL) cholesterol. However, we now know that these fats also lower good (HDL) cholesterol. So who needs them? And they make you just as fat as any other fat! I cringe every time I hear some misguided person say, "Oh, it's vegetable oil. It lowers cholesterol. It's good for you." In addition, polyunsaturated fats, such as corn oil, have been shown to produce tumors in laboratory rats.

What about "trans" fats? These are, in essence, synthetic brothers to saturated fats. Although technically they are unsaturated, they appear to have the same effect on our bodies as saturated fats. They are found in partially hydrogenated oil, and tend to be used in chips, crackers, cookies, granola bars, some cereals, and in many fried and fast foods.

Trans fats are also found in margarine. Up until recently margarine was touted as a healthier option to butter. But we now know that margarine may be even worse for your health than butter. Not only do trans fats such as in margarine tend to increase bad (LDL) cholesterol, just like butter they may decrease good (LDL) cholesterol.

What's the bottom line? Keep your fat intake low, period. If you're a woman, consume no more than 25 grams a day while you're losing weight, and if you're a man, no more than 40 grams a day.

When reading food labels, which will be discussed later, look for the *total fat grams per serving*. After you reach your goal—on the days when you are allowed to eat anything you want—for health reasons you might want to stick to monounsaturated fats. That will depend upon your cholesterol level and your doctor's advice.

Omega 3 Fatty Acids

For optimum health and prevention of atherosclerosis, rheumatoid arthritis, psoriasis, and other inflammatory conditions, as well as prevention of blood clots, it's a good idea to include a certain amount of omega 3 fatty acids in your diet. There are no specific recommended amounts of this nutrient, but you will note that every so often I include fish and soybean products high in omega 3 fatty acids.

CHOLESTEROL—IT'S NOT A FAT

You read that right. Cholesterol is *not* a fat but a fatlike, waxy substance that is produced in the liver naturally and obtained in the diet as well. An overabundance of cholesterol in your bloodstream can cause major problems to your health because it can clog your arteries.

When it comes to producing damaging blood cholesterol, the most troublesome food is saturated fat. It's the saturated fat found in red meats such as beef, pork, lamb, and veal; organ meats such as kidneys, brains, and liver; poultry skin, full-fat dairy products; egg yolks; lunch meats such as salami, sausage, and bacon; hard shortenings such as lard, beef tallow, palm oil, and coconut oil; and trans-fatty acids that produce the artery-clogging bad (LDL) cholesterol. The foods that directly contain cholesterol, such as shrimp, squid, eel, crayfish, and conch, which are very low in fat, and other low-fat animal foods, such as white-meat poultry and low-fat fish, *are not the problem*. They are low in saturated fat. It is not the cholesterol in a food that produces artery-clogging cholesterol in the blood, but the saturated fat. Get that straight—once and for all.

Is cholesterol a total enemy to the human body? Not at all. In fact, it is a necessary component. Our brain, liver, blood, nerve linings, and cell membranes are partially formed of cholesterol. In addition, cholesterol helps to form vitamin D and bile, as well as our adrenal and sex hormones. But the body does not need an outside source to get cholesterol because it naturally produces its own.

Cholesterol divides into two categories: "bad" cholesterol, which is labeled low-density lipoprotein, or LDL, and "good" cholesterol, which is labeled high-density lipoprotein, or HDL. The bad cholesterol can clog arteries by depositing itself on the arterial walls and forming plaque. When this happens, the blood cannot flow freely to and from the heart, causing many problems, including a potential heart attack.

"Good" cholesterol functions in the opposite manner. It unclogs your arteries by removing bad cholesterol from your tissues and taking it to your liver for elimination.

So when you ask, "Do I have high cholesterol?" what you're really asking is, "Do I have the right proportion of good to bad cholesterol?" To simplify the matter, however, most people with a problem simply say "My cholesterol level is high." What they mean is, "My bad cholesterol is too high." They should only be so lucky as to have a high good cholesterol level.

How do you find out your HDL to LDL ratio? You must take what is called a fractionated cholesterol test that yields an index. The lower your index, the lower your risk of heart attack. An index of 4 or lower is considered safe and healthy. First, find out your total cholesterol count, and then find out how the count breaks down into HDL and LDL. Then figure out your index. I'll show you how by doing mine.

As of this writing, my total cholesterol is 176. My HDL is 54, and my LDL is 122. I divide my total cholesterol count, which is 176, by my good cholesterol, which is 54. The index turns out to be 3.25. Since 4 would be perfectly fine, and mine is lower, I'm in great shape. I don't worry about eating low-fat, high-cholesterol foods such as shrimp—which I love and eat plenty of anyway—because they do not tend to produce cholesterol; in addition, on my free eating days, if I feel like it, I have a juicy red steak.

All foods high in cholesterol-producing fat are already forbidden in your diet while losing weight because fat is fat and it makes you fat. But what about cholesterol-containing foods in this diet? The consensus of the medical community is that one should consume 300 milligrams or less of cholesterol in the daily diet, just to be on the safe side—even though it is not cholesterol in food but saturated fat that is the main "maker" of artery-clogging blood cholesterol. Eating foods that have no cholesterol but that are high in saturated fat would be the biggest mistake you could make if you are concerned with heart disease.

Fatty Food No-No's Until You Reach Your Goal

All of the following foods have an average of 10 grams (or more) for a very small serving. These are off-limits when you are on your weight-loss diet:

butter, margarine, oil of any kind (except for canola on
    occasion), lard, fat of any kind
mayonnaise, fat-containing salad dressings
peanut butter
nuts, seeds
"chips" (potato, corn, etc.)
doughnuts, croissants
olives, avocados
fat-containing ice cream, sour cream, cream cheese, cookies,
    cake
dairy products over 1 percent fat
beef, pork, veal, bacon

Note: In general, even 1 percent fat products should give way to nonfat; however, when needed to fulfill your daily fat allowance, you can indulge—you will see this in the meal plans.

Don't worry about cooking without the fat or oil. There's a whole chapter coming up next on how to do that.

A Sample List of Forbidden Fatty Foods

Fast-food hamburgers, beef, chicken, fish, and Mexican food or sandwiches are off the OK list. Just take a look at how much fat they contain.

Food Product	Fat Grams
Burger King whopper	36
Burger King whopper with cheese	45
Burger King double whopper	52
Burger King double whopper with cheese	62
Arby's super roast beef sandwich	28
McDonald's Sausage McMuffin with egg	27.4
Arby's turkey sandwich	24
Burger King ham and cheese sandwich	24
Hot dog	15
4 ounces fast-food chicken thigh	19
4 ounces fast-food chicken drumstick	16
4 ounces fast-food chicken breast	15
Arthur Treacher's fried fish	19.7
Arthur Treacher's fish sandwich	19.2
Corn dog	16
Jack in the Box super taco	17
Taco Bell burrito	20
4 ounces refried beans with sausage	32

Subway Subs (6 inch)	Fat Grams
Ham and cheese	9
Turkey	9
Veggies and cheese	9
Roast beef	12
Steak and cheese	13
Cold cut combo	22
Tuna salad with mayo	49

Fast-Food Potato Dishes	Fat Grams
Burger King French fries	22
Wendy's baked potato with cheese	24

Fast-Food Dessert Products	Fat Grams
Dairy Queen banana split	15
Large Dairy Queen ice cream dipped in chocolate	20

Fatty Snacks (4 ounces)	Fat Grams
3 oil-roasted almonds	91
Dry-roasted almonds	71
Oil-roasted mixed nuts	81
Dry-roasted mixed nuts	70
Tortilla chips	9
Potato chips	10

PROTEIN: A MINIMUM OF 45 GRAMS A DAY, 55 FOR MEN

On this diet, you will get most of your fat from your required amount of low-fat protein. Don't worry, I'm not going to ask you to count protein grams, either. I've done the work for you. However, when you begin to plan your own eating program, you'll want to know about protein grams.

Why is protein important for good health? Indeed, protein is what is called the "building blocks" of the body. Muscle is made of protein. Protein is the essential repair material for the body. The internal organs, skin, hair, nails, and blood consist mainly of protein. Protein also affects production of the hormones that control metabolism, growth, and sexual development. Protein also helps to regulate the acid-alkaline balance of the blood and tissues, as well as control the body's water balance.

Protein consists of twenty-two elements called amino acids. The human body is capable of producing fourteen of these amino acids, and does not need food or any outside source for help. However, the remaining eight amino acids must be obtained from specific foods. The foods containing these eight essential amino acids are called *complete protein* foods and include poultry, red meat, fish, milk, milk products, eggs, or a combination of rice and beans, or corn and milk. The combinations work even if you eat them in the same week.

Your body needs a bare minimum of about 45 grams of protein a day if you are a woman and 55 if you are a man. However, if you're eating low-fat protein, you can consume a gram of protein for a pound of body weight. You can do this for several reasons. First, not all of your protein will be complete protein. Even though the protein count for a given day seems high (there is protein in nearly every food, even pears, oatmeal, and onions), it will not all be complete protein. Second, the protein is low in fat and will not make you fat. Third, although there is no proof, many people find that a little extra protein helps kick up the metabolism and make you burn more fat. Fourth, if you work out with weights, your body tends to crave more protein. Again there's no proof of this, but it's my experience and that of many exercise experts.

You will note that the meal plans here vary in daily protein intake. Feel free to make substitutions if you think the protein is too high or low for you; just remember to keep your fat grams and other foods within the food guidelines.

Where will you get your protein? You'll get it from white-meat poultry, fish, beans, and tofu.

Low-Fat Sources of Protein

All poultry is without skin and cooked without fat. I list the fat grams for your convenience.

Poultry (4 ounces cooked)	Grams of Fat	Grams of Protein
Turkey breast	1	34
Turkey drumstick	4.5	33
Turkey thigh	5	31
Chicken breast	4.5	35
Chicken drumstick	6.8	37
Chicken thigh	5	31

Fish (4 ounces cooked)	Grams of Fat	Grams of Protein
Mahimahi (dolphin fish)	0.8	20.8
Haddock	1	23
Cod	1	26
Abalone	1	16
Sole	1	19
Pike	1	25
Scallops	1	26
Tuna in water	1	34
Squid	1.8	20
Flounder	2.3	34
Red snapper	2.3	26
Sea bass	3.4	25
Halibut	4	31
Trout	4	30

Other Sources of Protein	Grams of Fat	Grams of Protein
4 ounces low-fat yogurt	2	6
4 ounces nonfat yogurt	0	7
8 ounces 1% milk	3	8
8 ounces skim milk	1	8
4 ounces (½ cup) 1% cottage cheese	1	14
2 tablespoons nonfat cream cheese	0	2
1½ slices (1½ ounces) nonfat cheese	0	9
½ cup nonfat ice cream	0	2
3 egg whites	1	9
½ cup beans*	1	9
½ cup soft tofu*	6	10
½ cup firm tofu*	11	19

* Vegetarian sources of protein.

What About Soy Products?

The latest research into soy foods has them at the top of the list with overall super healthy foods. In fact, it was recently shown that soy protein reduces LDL (bad cholesterol) when consumed in quantities of 50 grams a day.

Among the most wonderful qualities of soy products is the natural chemical phytoestrogen. The chemical is especially helpful to women entering menopause. This dietary source of estrogen has been shown to mitigate the symptoms of menopause, such as hot flashes, mood swings, and night sweats. I found this information especially important, since so many women are leery of hormone replacement. In fact, many women tell me the soy products (I've included some of my favorite recipes here) help with the symptoms mentioned above.

The way I see it, using soy foods may be one way to manage menopause with food instead of using medicine. Tiffany Middendorf, who wrote the foreword to this book, indicates that the recommendations are 1 cup of soy milk or ½ cup tofu for women approaching menopause. She points out that Asians (who eat a lot of soy products) don't even have a word for "hot flash."

The good news about soy products is they are all now available in low- and even nonfat varieties. But even those soy products with fat left in are beneficial to health, since the fat present in soy resembles omega 3 fat in fish (discussed on page 52). This fat acts somewhat as a blood thinner. Also, as a protein, soy is less damaging than animal protein, which contains sulfur amino acids. An overabundance of these can cause the body to draw calcium from the bones and excrete it in the urine. For this reason, many nutritional experts feel that soy rates above dairy products and even lean meats.

Soy products include soy milk, tofu (a curdled compressed soy milk that comes in firm and soft varieties, firm being more condensed), tempeh (made from condensed, fermented soybeans), and soy flour (made from ground soybeans). Miso (a paste made from fermented soybeans and rice or barley) is advised for occasional use only due to its high sodium content. As mentioned above, all of these products come in low- and many even in nonfat varieties.

WHAT ARE CARBOHYDRATES?

Carbohydrates divide into two categories: simple and complex. These categories themselves divide into simple processed or "refined" and simple unprocessed.

The simple processed or refined carbohydrates are sugars found as white bread, sourdough bread, sugar candy, syrup, pie, cookies, cake, honey, jam, jelly, soda, sweet rolls—any sugar product, which includes sucrose, glucose, dextrose, fructose, maltose, sorbitol, and xylitol. The simple unprocessed carbohydrates are fruit.

The complex carbohydrates divide into two categories: limited (bread, cereal, pasta, rice, corn, peas, beets, and potatoes) and unlimited (all other vegetables). Much more about that later; for now, let's talk about the function of carbohydrates.

It is carbohydrates that supply energy to both your body and your brain. Simple carbohydrates such as fruit provide an immediate energy burst and it ends there, while complex carbohydrates provide gradually released energy that can last for hours.

Eat 2 to 4 Fruits a Day; Occasional Refined Carbohydrates Allowed

Your source of simple unprocessed or unrefined carbohydrates will be fruit. Fruit supplies your body with much-needed vitamins and fiber and gives you a quick energy burst. It's better not to eat fruit on an empty stomach, however, because you may experience an energy letdown. Better to eat fruit after at least a small snack of complex carbohydrates.

But what's wrong with eating simple processed carbohydrates, such as white bread, sourdough bread, sugar candy, syrup, pie, cookies, cake, honey, jam, jelly, soda, sweet rolls, or sugar products? When you eat these foods, glucose is pumped into your bloodstream at such a rapid speed that it quickly elevates your insulin level. When this happens, the enzyme (hormone-sensitive lipase) responsible for pulling fat from your fat cells is hindered from its work. Fat is trapped in your fat cells, and your body is forced to burn more carbohydrates and less fat. In essence, your weight-loss efforts are hindered. In addition, your appetite is stimulated and it's that much harder to keep to your diet!

If that is the case, why don't I forbid any sugary foods? Because you may be like me and need an occasional sweet to prevent you from going off your diet completely and eating a worse food enemy, fat. For this reason, if you can handle it, I allow you to occasionally indulge in a low-fat or nonfat sugary treat. You are allowed, from time to time, to substitute a fruit or a limited complex carbohydrate for a sugary treat. I've worked these options into your meal plans, but note that they are options. You don't have to use them.

What about artificial sweeteners and the no-calorie drinks containing them? The studies of artificial sweeteners continue, for some medical authorities feel they are potential health risks. I used to consume loads of artificial sweeteners and sodas, but now I keep them to a minimum. You'll have to make your own choice here.

What about juice? When fruit is processed into juice, it behaves exactly like a sugar and will hinder your body's ability to burn fat the same way sugar does. Believe it or not, it's true, so stick to the fruit! What's more, the fruit has fiber and bulk, and won't give you as much of an energy burst and concomitant letdown.

Following are some serving sizes for fruits:

One Serving Equals

1 large apple
1 small banana
1 medium pear
1 large kiwi
1 small mango
1 large nectarine
1 large orange
1 large peach
4 apricots
20 grapes
3 kumquats
3 persimmons
2 plums
2 fresh prunes
2 tangerines
15 large cherries
1 cup berries (any kind)
1 cup papaya
1½ cups strawberries
1½ cups watermelon cubes
½ cantaloupe
½ grapefruit
¼ large pineapple
½ large plantain
4 ounces nonfat ice cream
¼ honeydew melon
1 ounce raisins or figs
4-ounce can of fruit, unsweetened, in its own juice (no more than 1 serving a day)
½ cup juice (no more than 1 serving a day to replace a fruit, but actual fruit is *always* better than juice)
100 calories nonfat cake, hard candy, cookies
100 calories' worth of fruit-based jam or jelly

Nonfat or Sugar-Free Foods

You have to really be careful about sugar-free foods because they may be loaded with fat, and most of the calories are in fat, not sugar. But what about fat-free foods? Watch out for an over-abundance of sugar because sugar, as discussed earlier, can hinder your body's ability to burn fat.

Nonfat foods such as nonfat ice cream, cottage cheese, or cream cheese are not necessarily low in calories. Although your meal plan strictly limits the amount of these products you can eat, when they are not restricted some people tend to overindulge, thinking, "Well, they are fat free so I can't get fat." They might consume a gallon of nonfat ice cream in a couple of days or a box of nonfat cookies. But these items may be loaded with sugar and hinder fat burning, as discussed above. In addition, the calories add up, and little or no weight loss is realized—and in some cases, weight gain occurs. I'm not asking you to stay away from nonfat or no-sugar foods. Just be alert so you can use them wisely.

COMPLEX CARBOHYDRATES: LIMITED AND UNLIMITED

Complex carbohydrates divide into two groups: limited and unlimited. The limited ones are restricted because, although they are low in fat or have no fat, they have enough calories per serving to matter if you ate them in unlimited quantities. The unlimited complex carbohydrates are allowed in abundance because they don't contain enough calories to hinder your weight loss, no matter how much of them you eat.

Caloric density is the number of calories per weight of a particular food. We want to keep our calories low in order to lose weight, so the foods that are *low in caloric density* are the best bargain because they fill your stomach without causing you to eat too many calories.

Foods low in caloric density are found in both limited and unlimited categories. Potatoes, sweet potatoes, yams, pasta, rice, and hot cereals are filling foods that are low in calories, as opposed to bread and cold cereals, which are light and don't fill up your stomach as quickly. Although calories are not the issue, broccoli and cauliflower are examples of filling foods, as opposed to lettuce or escarole.

How does food make us feel full, anyway? Since the stomach holds a maximum of 2 pounds of food, you can only eat so much at one sitting. Suppose you are in that "eat until I'm stuffed" mood. Choose low-caloric-density foods for your meal: hot cereal, potatoes or pasta, cauliflower, broccoli, tomatoes, carrots, red peppers, cucumbers, and so on to accompany your allowed protein. You will be able to put 2 pounds' worth of food in your stomach that way without going over your food allotment. If, on the other hand, you try to fill up on cereal—cornflakes, for example, which contain 380 calories for every 3.5 ounces—you would have to eat about 3,800 calories to consume 2 pounds of food to fill your stomach.

If you tried to fill up on whole wheat bread, you would have to eat the whole loaf at 45 calories a slice—and the calories would add up to 1,600. Still your stomach would have only 1 pound of food in it and you would not feel full. On the other hand, if you ate a cup each of broccoli, cauliflower, carrots, and pasta, you would be full—and what's more, you would have only consumed about 400 calories! Of course, you would not be so foolish as to want to eat 2 pounds of cornflakes or a whole loaf of whole wheat bread, but suffice it to say that if you're really hungry and want that full feeling, stick to the "heavier" foods that are low in caloric density.

Does this mean that we should never eat whole wheat bread or lightweight foods such as cereal? Of course not. But on those days when you're really hungry, choose the heavier, low-caloric-density foods, or at least use the unlimited ones to supplement your meal. All of the "before and after" women in Chapter 2 told me they do this, and I do it all the time.

Eat 5 to 7 Limited Complex Carbohydrates (8 to 10 for Men)

Now let's talk about the *limited complex carbohydrates.* Why limit anything as long as it's low in fat? Because if you want to lose weight, although high-fat foods are much worse for you than low-fat foods, you will not lose weight if you eat more calories than you burn, and you could even gain weight. So, women should eat six to eight (eight to eleven for men) servings of limited complex carbohydrates a day: bread, whole wheat, rye, or pumpernickel; grains; cereal; rice; pasta; corn; beans; peas; beets; lentils; and potatoes. For the limited complex carbohydrates, one portion is:

Breads, Cereals, Grains

½ bagel
2 slices light bread
1 English muffin
8 low- or nonfat crackers
4 rice cakes
1 pita bread
¾ cup cold cereal (dry)
1 ounce hot cereal (before cooking)
⅔ cup cooked pasta
⅔ cup cooked rice
½ cup cooked barley
1 ounce pretzels or 1 "serving" size
100 calories worth of non- or low-fat cake, cookies, etc.
   (one "serving" of package)
3 cups popcorn, made with no oil

Vegetables

1 baked potato
¾ cup Jerusalem artichoke
1 small sweet potato or yam

1 cup corn kernels
1 large corn on the cob
½ cup beans or lentils of any kind (used also as protein)
1 cup peas of any kind
1 cup beets
1 cup acorn (winter) squash

Note: Consumption of vegetable juices is limited. You can have two 6-ounce servings a day. This is because some people might drink four quarts of vegetable juice a day, and then the calories add up. Also, I want you to get the bulk (fiber) from real vegetables.

Can Pasta Make You Fat?

Let's clear up a myth once and for all. Not too long ago there was a *New York Times* article that scared pasta lovers half to death. It said that pasta can make you fat! Apparently, some researchers feel that when pasta is consumed, the insulin level rises, and in turn the body converts the calories into fat.* The Pritikin Longevity Center and many other nutritional groups have since decried the article as a "mishmash" of information.

The good news is that pasta will not make you fat. The first mistake in the article was to not differentiate between refined or processed carbohydrates, mainly sugars, and unrefined complex carbohydrates, such as pasta—especially when the pasta is cooked al dente. The fact is, unrefined complex carbohydrates such as pasta do not cause the same insulin response as do refined complex carbohydrates. In fact, when pasta is consumed, a very mild insulin response occurs and a minimum amount of body fat is produced and stored. In discussing this issue, *Vantage Point*, the newsletter of The Pritikin Longevity Center, cites a study in which seventy-two men and women followed a diet rich in unrefined carbohydrates such as pasta, and

*Molly O'Neill, "So It May Be True After All: Pasta Makes You Fat." *New York Times*, February 6, 1996, pp. 1A, C6; "Pasta's Fattening?" Pritikin *Vantage Point*, May 1995, pp. 1–3.

their insulin *dropped* on an average of 32 percent. For your information, The Pritikin Longevity Center specifically recommends the following foods as having a low glycemic response, and hence a low fat production and storage response: whole-grain cereals, especially oatmeal; corn, barley, brown rice; beans; peas, lentils, garbanzos; vegetables; pastas, preferably al dente and whole-grain; yams, sweet potatoes, and boiled new potatoes; and fresh whole raw fruit.

Eat 6 to Unlimited Amounts of Unlimited Complex Carbohydrates

Now what about the *unlimited complex carbohydrates* and why are they unlimited? The answer is simple: they don't contain enough calories to hinder weight loss, no matter how much you eat of them. But note, there is a minimum, and my minimum is higher than the three to five servings per day guideline of the USDA. Why? If you don't fill up on these foods, you'll feel hungry and may want to overeat the limited foods, or worse, you'll be tempted to indulge in the forbidden foods. Therefore, eat six to unlimited amounts of most vegetables daily. One serving equals any vegetable, except for those listed in the limited complex category. For optimum health, be sure to eat dark green or yellow-orange vegetables at least once a day. This would be almost impossible not to do on this plan because, as you will quickly note, most of the vegetables are those colors. But I say this just in case you decide to eat ten cups of mushrooms and onions at the expense of all other vegetables!

1 Serving = ½ Cup Cooked or 1 Cup Raw

    Asparagus
    Broccoli
    Brussels sprouts
    Cabbage, Chinese cabbage
    Cauliflower

Carrots
Celery
Chicory
Collard greens
Cucumber
Eggplant
Frozen mixed vegetables
Endive
Escarole
Kale
Leeks
Lettuce
Mushrooms
Green or yellow beans
Okra
Onions
Parsnips
Peppers, green or red
Radishes
Rutabagas
Shallots
Spinach
Sprouts
Squash (summer or zucchini)
Tomatoes
Turnips

YOUR REQUIRED DAILY FIBER

Luckily, you don't have to go out of your way and consume extra food in order to consume your healthful 30 grams of daily fiber. You'll naturally get your fiber in fruit (there are 10 grams of fiber in a cup of strawberries, for example) and vegetables (there are 8 grams of fiber in a cup of broccoli). Cereals are also an excellent source of fiber. Check the cereal box for fiber grams. Kellogg's All-Bran and Bran Buds, and General Mills's

Fiber One have 10 to 14 grams of fiber per serving. You'll also get fiber from limited complex carbohydrates such as beans, peas, and lentils, which contain 16 grams of fiber per cup. Finally, be on the lookout for the highest fiber low-fat, low-calorie breads, such as Wonder Light Nine-Grain bread, which has only 1 gram of fat, 40 calories, and 6 grams of fiber. You might also want to try the delicious Beefsteak Light Soft Rye, which has only 35 calories a slice, 5 grams of fiber, and no fat. The only problem with this bread is that it's so delicious you may be tempted to eat the whole loaf during the course of a day. I've done it on more than one occasion! (There are many other excellent bread choices. Be sure to read the labels, and be aware that if the loaf is wheat, it must be whole wheat. If it just says "wheat," it's refined white bread!)

But why is fiber so important? Not only does it help with elimination and prevention of disease, it helps remove fat from the body! Yes. As fiber exits your body through elimination, some of the fat in your digestive system clings to the rough surface of the fiber and pulls the fat along with it. In this sense, fiber behaves as a "fat vacuum."

Fiber falls into two categories: *soluble fiber,* which is found in oat bran, psyllium, fresh fruits and vegetables, and legumes, and *insoluble fiber,* which is found in whole wheat, whole grains, celery, corn, corn bran, green beans, green leafy vegetables, potato skins, and brown rice. Soluble fiber can be digested by the body when consumed. It helps to lower blood sugar and cholesterol levels. Insoluble fiber cannot be digested by the body. About 15 percent of a food with this type of fiber is automatically eliminated, and in that sense the calorie count to these foods is really 15 percent less than you think. Insoluble fiber also provides the stool with needed volume and helps prevent constipation and colon or rectal cancer.

VITAMINS AND MINERALS AND CANCER-PREVENTION FOODS

If you follow the diet in this book, you will be getting all your required vitamins and minerals from real food. It is always best to get your vitamins and minerals from real food, but if you are in doubt, consult your nutritionist for a vitamin and mineral supplement. Whatever you do, don't start taking megadoses of vitamins, minerals, and herbal products without your doctor's okay. Recent research has indicated that such intake can be toxic!

In any case, know that eating a diet high in beta-carotene (found in apricots, cantaloupe, carrots, sweet potatoes, and dark green vegetables) helps prevent skin cancer (melanoma), breast cancer, and lung cancer. As beta-carotene is converted to vitamin A in the digestive system, it "neutralizes" what are called free radicals (agents that can make the body vulnerable to cancer).

In addition, eating what are called the cruciferous vegetables (cabbage family, such as broccoli, cauliflower, and Brussels sprouts) helps prevent colon cancer. Fruits and vegetables high in vitamin C help prevent all kinds of cancer by causing your body to produce flavonoids—antioxidants that slow down a cancerous malignancy.

THE MINERALS SODIUM AND CALCIUM

Many people don't realize it, but sodium is a needed mineral, required by the body to regulate body fluids and maintain the acid-alkali balance of the blood. If you have too little sodium in your system, your muscles will cramp and even shrink because sodium is responsible for muscle contraction. On the other hand, overconsumption of salt causes problems of water retention.

Sodium holds about fifty times its weight in water. When you consume too much sodium, your body temporarily retains excess water, and since water weighs a pound a quart, the scale goes up. In addition, you look and feel bloated. But the weight gain is temporary. As soon as you return to moderate sodium intake, the water is eliminated. There's a big difference between a temporary water weight gain and a fat weight gain that is not temporary—the latter takes much more effort to lose.

Most medical authorities agree that a healthy daily sodium intake is 1,500 to 2,500 milligrams per day, unless of course, you suffer from high blood pressure and your doctor makes a specific recommendation. (The Pritikin Longevity Center recommends that you not go over 1,600 milligrams per day.) Just in case you're wondering, there are 2,000 milligrams of sodium in a teaspoon of salt. A few good shakes of the salt shaker can easily add up to 500 or more milligrams of salt, so be aware!

There are other issues related to sodium. Recent research indicates that 1 teaspoon of salt a day can equate to 1 percent loss of skeletal bone mass.

Frankly, I don't think about my sodium intake. I don't have high blood pressure—in fact, it's rather low. In addition, my bone density is *double* the density of women my age because I work out with weights. I have enough trouble worrying about fat. I don't care if I retain water! When I have a photo shoot or TV appearance, then I keep my sodium low. In fact, I regularly add at least ¼ teaspoon of salt per serving to most meal plans, but in general I've kept the sodium low in the recipes so you have the option of adding it yourself.

How much sodium is found in various foods? There are about 500 milligrams of sodium in ¼ teaspoon of regular table salt, and about 275 in "lite" salt. You will notice that from time to time I include an optional ¼ teaspoon of salt in a recipe. If you don't have a blood pressure problem, feel free to use the salt. Otherwise use the spice substitutes.

Canned foods always are very high in sodium, unless they are specifically billed as reduced sodium. For example, one serving of a canned soup usually contains 900 milligrams of sodium. A serving of canned string beans has about 600 milligrams of sodium, but frozen or fresh string beans have less than 50 milligrams a serving.

As for calcium, a deficiency can contribute to bone density loss, or osteoporosis. It's a good idea to follow the recommendations of most doctors and consume a minimum of 1,200 to 1,500 milligrams of calcium daily. This means you should eat two to three dairy foods per day for your calcium requirement.

The following list will give you an idea of how much calcium is found in various foods.

Food Item	Calcium Content (milligrams)
8 ounces skim milk	302
8 ounces 1% milk	300
8 ounces calcium-fortified orange juice	300
4 ounces firm tofu	258
2 ounces nonfat cheese	255
4 ounces low-fat yogurt	200
4 ounces ocean perch	156
4 ounces soft tofu	130
½ cup cooked turnip greens	90
½ cup cooked broccoli	89
½ cup soybeans	88
4 ounces (½ cup) nonfat cottage cheese	87
½ cup cooked collard greens	74
½ cup cooked dandelion greens	73
4 ounces (½ cup) 1% cottage cheese	69
½ cup navy beans	64
½ cup cooked mustard greens	52
½ cup cooked kale	47

Note: Cottage cheese is not considered as good a calcium source as other dairy products. If you are not sure that you're getting enough calcium in your diet, see your doctor about taking a supplement. You can get much of your calcium requirement from your dairy requirement. Note: Women who are not in menopause can have 800–1,000 milligrams of calcium but women in menopause need about 1,500 milligrams.

As you may have noticed, you can get much of your calcium from your dairy allowance. Note that on occasion—say, once a week—you can substitute a nonfat ice cream for a dairy requirement.

Eat 2 to 3 dairy servings per day.

One Serving Equals

1 glass of skim or 1% milk
8 ounces nonfat or 1% yogurt
4 ounces nonfat or 1% cottage cheese

One Serving Equals (*cont.*)

2 tablespoons nonfat or 1% cream cheese
1½ slices nonfat cheese
½ cup nonfat ice cream

I get my daily calcium by putting 1% or skim milk in my coffee and on cold cereal, and by eating 1% or nonfat cottage cheese or yogurt.

HOW TO READ FOOD LABELS

Nutrition Facts

Serving Size ½ cup (54 g)
(About 1 cup cooked)
Servings Per Container about 7

Amount Per Serving

Calories 190	Calories from Fat 15

	% Daily Value *
Total Fat 1.5 g	**2**%
Saturated Fat 0 g	**0**%
Cholesterol 0 mg	**0**%
Sodium 20 mg	**1**%
Total Carbohydrate 42 g	**14**%
Dietary Fiber 2 g	**8**%
Sugars 0 g	
Protein 4 g	

Vitamin A 0%	Vitamin C 0%
Calcium 0%	Iron 2%

* Percent Daily Values are based on a 2,000 calorie diet. Your daily values may be higher or lower depending on your calorie needs:

		Calories:	2,000	2,500
Total Fat	Less than		65 g	80 g
Sat Fat	Less than		20 g	25 g
Cholesterol	Less than		300 mg	300 mg
Sodium	Less than		2,400 mg	2,400 mg
Total Carbohydrate			300 g	375 g
Dietary Fiber			25 g	30 g

INGREDIENTS: PRECOOKED LONG GRAIN BROWN RICE.

The new food labels are easy to read. You can quickly tell how many grams of fat there are in a serving. You can also tell how many grams of protein you are getting, how many calories per serving, and how much fiber. These factors will be your main concerns. For further information, you'll learn specifically how much saturated fat and how much cholesterol is found in the food. You'll also learn how much sugar, sodium, and calcium and vitamins are contained in the food.

Before we talk about the helpful aspects of food labels, however, first let me tell you what to ignore—and why. The column to the right, "% Daily Value," and the two boxes at the very bottom of the label are useless information because they are based on the assumption that you are going to consume a diet of 30 percent fat—or simply put, about twice the amount of fat grams you are consuming. In addition, this information assumes that you are going to eat 2,000 calories a day.

Now let's talk about how to use the information on the food label for your benefit. Look at the "Nutrition Facts" section and note the serving size. In this case it is ½ cup raw brown rice, 1 cup cooked. You are given extra information, "Servings Per Container," and note that there are seven servings per container. Why do you care? If you're like me, you sometimes eat the whole box of something. Then you can quickly figure out the damage you've done by multiplying everything by the serving size. But I don't think you're in danger of going hog wild over brown rice. In fact, I think 1 cup cooked—their serving—will be quite satisfying.

Now look at the next section, "Amount Per Serving." First note the calories section. It says there are 190 calories in the cup of cooked brown rice. Not bad because rice is quite filling. But wait a minute; the label tells me calories from fat. Do I care? No. But if you did care, you would quickly do your figuring and discover that the rice has only 7 percent fat. Nice to know. But more important is what is found the next line down, "Total Fat." It says 1.5 grams! So by eating the rice, which is just over one of your six to eight servings of limited complex carbohydrates, you consume only 1.5 of your allowed 20 to 25 grams of fat.

The next column down is "Cholesterol." Here you discover that the rice has no cholesterol. Going down the label, the next column, "Sodium," tells you that there are only 20 milligrams of sodium in the rice—very low— about 1 percent of your maximum daily allowance even on this eating plan.

Continuing down the label, the next line reads "Total Carbohydrate." It says 42 grams. This is of no concern to you, since the large majority of your diet is carbohydrates. You don't have to worry about limiting them, except in the cases I've already explained.

The next line reads "Dietary Fiber." Note that there are 2 grams of dietary fiber in the rice. So you've gotten two out of thirty grams for your daily requirement of fiber. Moving down the label, we come to the line that reads "Sugars." You quickly see that there are no sugars in the rice. Good, because you want to keep your sugars low. Continuing down the label, finally, we get to the last line that concerns us: "Protein." There are 4 grams of protein in the rice. This could be counted as full protein as long as you eat it with, say, a half cup of beans (which in itself would add another 8 grams of protein), bringing you up to 12 grams of complete protein. Not bad, and look how low in fat your food intake would be for fulfilling part of your protein requirement.

There's yet another section of the food label that is of interest: the ingredients list, found at the very bottom of the label. Here, the contents of the package are listed in relation to each other. In the case of the rice, you don't learn much because, as you will note, all it says is "Precooked Long Grain Brown Rice." But the labels of other food products that consist of a variety of ingredients can be informative for one reason: food manufacturers are required to list the ingredients in *the order of amount*. In other words, they must list the food that is contained in the package in the greatest amount first, and so on.

How can this help you? A certain cereal may have listed: whole oat flour, sugar, modified cornstarch, corn syrup, dextrose, wheat starch, salt. . . . What do you learn? You discover that there's an awful lot of sugar in the food. You've noted that not only is plain sugar listed as the second ingredient but it occurs again not much later down the line as corn syrup and dextrose. Of course, you don't have to depend upon the ingredients list to know this. Had you read the nutrition label for this product, you would have quickly found out that the cereal has 13 grams of sugars and only 11 grams of other carbohydrates.

Wait a minute. Didn't the ingredients list place whole oat flour—a nonsugar carbohydrate—first and wouldn't this imply that there should be more grams of "other carbohydrates" than sugar? No. Not when you realize that if added up, the sugar, corn syrup, and dextrose can easily add up to more than the whole oat flour! That's why the new food labels are so wonderful—they force the food manufacturers to tell all. No more fooling the consumer.

Labels That Say 98% Fat Free—or Some Such Thing

Beware of food labels that disguise the true fat content of a given item. For example, a ground turkey label may say "93% fat free" when in reality the turkey gets 45 percent of its calories from fat and should read "55 percent fat free." You are led to believe that only 7 percent of the turkey is fat. How can they get away with this?

They do it by basing their claim on the total weight of the product rather than on the total calorie count. For instance, a serving of the turkey is 3.5 ounces. There are 7 grams of fat in the turkey. Seven grams is only 7 percent of the weight of the serving of turkey, 3.5 ounces. But if you figure it out by calorie, you get a different picture.

Seven grams of fat at 9 calories a gram equals 63 calories of fat. How much is 63 divided by the total calorie count, which is 140? The answer is 45 percent. So we see that the turkey is made up of 45 percent fat. The label should have read "55% fat free." Now that's a horse of a different color.

But you wouldn't have been fooled anyway. Chances are, you would realize that white meat, skinned turkey, as listed in your low-fat protein food source list, has only 2 grams of fat for 4 ounces and so is a better deal than the ground turkey. And by the way, don't bother with any protein source that is "ground." You can be sure that most manufacturers are going to use "filler fat" to get their top dollar for a product. Fat is cheap. Meat is expensive. Don't be fooled.

WHAT ABOUT WATER?

Water keeps the skin looking young because it plumps out sagging skin. It also cleanses the inner body. In addition, contrary to what you might think, drinking lots of water does not cause you to retain water. It ensures that you will not retain water because it flushes the excess sodium out of your system. But perhaps the most important thing to know about water is, if your body is dehydrated, you will think you are hungry when really all you may need is some water. Most foods are more than 70 percent water. In an effort to force you to give it water, knowing that you don't drink water, your body may lead you to food. To ensure younger-looking skin, good health, and control of your appetite, you should drink six to eight 8-ounce glasses of water a day. If you hate water, put a splash of lemon or orange juice in the water.

Why do we need so much water? More than half of our body weight is water. We could live for a month without eating, but we could survive only a few days without water, because the human body loses three quarts of water per day through perspiration and excretion. (Our bodies cannot store excess water for any length of time, the way they store excess food.)

Water is the basis of all body fluids, including digestive juices, blood, urine, lymph secretions, and perspiration. It is the primary carrier of nutrients throughout the body, and is involved in nearly every body function, including absorption and digestion, excretion, circulation, lubrication, and regulation of body temperature.

CAFFEINE

Caffeine is best kept in moderation. Although some studies indicate that it is good for the heart when consumed in moderate amounts, and clearly it provides an energy boost, other studies indicate that it can be bad for the heart, especially in excess. In addition, caffeine can cause fibrocystic breast tissue, stress, decreased blood flow to the brain, nausea, insomnia, fast pulse, increased need to urinate, raised cholesterol levels, and even decreased ability to absorb calcium.

Caffeine is found in food items other than coffee. Going from most to least per cup, a cup of brewed coffee has about 125 milligrams of caffeine, while instant coffee has about 85. Most colas have about 50 milligrams a glass, and tea has about 35. Cocoa, the least of the lot, has approximately 35 milligrams of caffeine per cup.

I drink about three cups of brewed coffee a day, and I'd rather fight than switch. However, if I ever developed a fast heart rate or any other symptom that motivated me to stop drinking coffee, I would do it. But it would make me very sad.

ALCOHOL IN MODERATION

You will note that I have not included alcohol in any of the meal plans. However, if you wish to substitute one of your optional fruits or limited complex carbohydrates for an occasional drink, you may do so. For example, suppose it's a weekend night and you want two glasses of wine with your dinner. You've eaten only two pieces of fruit that day. Instead of having your fruit, you opt for the drinks. You are giving up healthful fiber and vitamins for controversial wine (some doctors feel a little is good for your health; others say to stay away). I wouldn't want you to do this more than once a week, preferably less when you are trying to lose weight.

What about the doctors who say one drink a day is fine?

They may be perfectly right, but I think drinking alcohol slows down your metabolism and encourages you to let down your guard. That is to say, you have a drink and you feel relaxed, so you say to yourself, "Oh, so what. I'll just eat this . . ." and before you know it, you've broken your diet. So better to forget the alcohol until you reach your goal—unless of course you know you can handle it.

What should you drink when you do drink alcohol? Stick to light beer, white or red wine, champagne, or drinks with alcohol and either juice (be careful, in bars they sometimes give you what seems like colored sugar water for orange juice), or diet soda. Otherwise, the calories add up quickly and you defeat your fat-loss plan. (Keep in mind that one serving of an alcoholic beverage is 4 ounces wine or champagne, 12 ounces of beer, or 1½ ounces of hard liquor.)

THE DAILY MEAL PLANS: COMPARISON WITH THE USDA'S FOOD PYRAMID

If you follow my meal plans, you will be basically following a modified version of the USDA's Food Pyramid and each day getting two to three servings of dairy, two to three servings of protein, two to four servings of fruit, and six to unlimited servings of vegetables.

In addition, you'll be getting the proper amount of calcium and fiber—and you'll be keeping your fat grams low (20 to 25 for women, 30 to 40 for men). And, you'll be keeping your saturated fat low because all fat is kept low. Your sodium and cholesterol will be kept well under the doctor's recommended amount. Calories in your meal plans will be low enough for you to lose weight, even though you eat a generous amount of unlimited complex carbohydrates!

Food Guide Pyramid
A Guide to Daily Food Choices

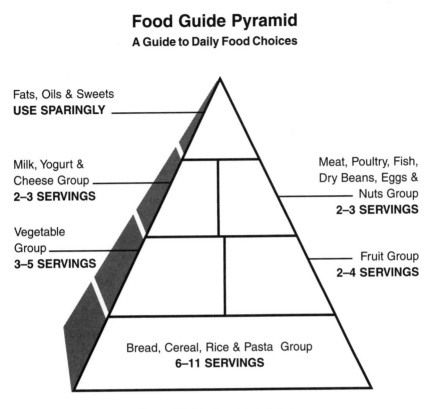

Fats, Oils & Sweets
USE SPARINGLY

Milk, Yogurt &
Cheese Group
2–3 SERVINGS

Meat, Poultry, Fish,
Dry Beans, Eggs &
Nuts Group
2–3 SERVINGS

Vegetable
Group
3–5 SERVINGS

Fruit Group
2–4 SERVINGS

Bread, Cereal, Rice & Pasta Group
6–11 SERVINGS

Source: U.S. Department of Agriculture

What's the difference between my diet plan and that of the USDA's Food Pyramid? The only difference is that I require you to eat six or more servings of vegetables, whereas the Food Pyramid requires a minimum of three servings. I feel that if you don't take advantage of the low-calorie high-density vegetables, you may feel hungry and be tempted to eat the wrong foods. Also note that because my bread, cereal, rice, and pasta group (limited complex carbohydrates) allows larger portions, you are allowed five rather than six as a minimum.

The Minimum or Maximum

I'm often asked, "Should I eat the minimum or maximum allowed?" In other words, since I have a choice of eating two or four fruit servings, do I eat two, three, or four? And since I have a choice of eating five, six, or seven limited complex carbohydrates, do I eat five, six, or seven?

Follow your body! On days when you are really hungry, don't deprive yourself—eat the maximum. On days when you could go either way, and you want to lose weight as soon as possible, pass up the optional maximum servings. Play it by ear. But whatever you do don't become so rigid with yourself that you hate your life and don't want to keep your diet. Easy does it. Everything in time.

It's the Big Picture That Counts

Okay. Now let's be realistic. Even the most astute dieters don't always eat exactly even the minimum amount of fruit, protein, dairy, et cetera. What happens then? Nothing. The body is an intelligent mechanism and it will balance itself out in the end.

If you use the food guidelines as a general rule, don't worry that on certain days your diet is not exactly following the plan. Think of it more as a weekly average than a rigid daily requirement.

HOW TO MAINTAIN YOUR WEIGHT LOSS FOR THE REST OF YOUR LIFE

Nice work! You Ate to Trim. You did indeed get it off. But how do you keep it off? Aside from maintaining a workout that will kick up your metabolism so that you burn more fat daily (as discussed in Chapter 10), how do you manage your eating so that you can enjoy your life without the constant threat of regaining the weight?

There are two plans. Plan A allows you to eat 15 to 20 percent more than you ate to lose the weight. For example, with this eating plan, you consume an average of about 1,500 calories a day. Once you reach your weight goal, you can add about 225 to 300 calories a day and still maintain your weight. You can have those calories in any kind of food at all, no matter how high the fat or sugar, but you will have to check with your doctor if it's "unhealthy" fat—especially if you have a heart condition.

Now let's talk about Plan B. This plan allows you to save up your extra eating for the end of the week. You can wait until the weekend, say, Saturday, and eat 1,575 to 2,100 extra calories, no matter what the fat or sugar content. Again, you must check with your doctor.

Which plan do I follow? Those of you who have read my previous workout books know that in my "diet" chapters, I always allow one day a week as a pig-out day. In fact once they reached their goal, I allowed my readers to eat anything they wanted all day long, one day a week. In the beginning, who knows, a person may consume 5,000 extra calories and all kinds of fat, sugar, and salt on that day. I clearly explained that I was counting on the fact that, like me, my readers would feel so sick the next day it would stop them from going that crazy on a regular basis.

For myself and many of my readers, this plan worked very well. We balance out and, in essence, really only consume about 2,000 calories of "naughty" foods on pig-out day. I am told by nutrition experts, however, that this plan can cause problems for some people who may not "balance out" and who may eat who knows how many calories and how much fat, sugar, and salt. Therefore, you should follow this important guideline: Do not consume more than the accumulated calorie amount of about 1,575 to 2,100 on the free eating day.

But that's not the only issue to consider. Nutrition experts agree that overeating in such a way once a week can cause fatigue, irritability, and constipation the next day and perhaps for a few days after. Well, it's true. I've had some of these symptoms the next day, but I don't care. For me it's sometimes worth it.

People who have heart conditions do not have the option of Plan B—at least not the full option. They cannot under any conditions consume unhealthy fats, sugars, and salt, especially in abundance. People with such conditions will have to ask their doctor which, if any, foods can be eaten in abundance on the once-a-week eating day. Chances are the doctor will recommend plan A instead, since it's a lot easier on the body.

Up until a few months ago, I always followed Plan B and it worked for me. In fact, it has been my life. I loved the fact that I had something to look forward to at the end of the week. But recently I tried plan A, and to my amazement, I liked it too. And to my surprise, I can do it. I always thought that if I ate one "forbidden" food, such as my favorite naughty food, Cheez-Its (and I'm talking about the full-fat kind), I would eat the whole huge box. Yes, I would still do that. But I have a trick. I buy the small box. The whole box is only 300 calories, and since I have no heart or blood pressure condition, I don't care about the fat or sodium. No problem.

The key is "know thyself." I know that I can cope with this one indiscretion for certain foods as long as there is no more left over to taunt me all day. If my extra food is going to be a bagel with lox and cream cheese, I know that I'm not as tempted to continue eating that all day, so I can have a few extra bagels and some leftover lox and cream cheese around. But what if you are the type of person who, even if there is no more of the forbidden food around, will go out and buy some more? Then for you, with your doctor's permission of course, Plan B is the thing.

What happens if you somehow go overboard—either on Plan A or Plan B—and find yourself, say, 3 to 5 pounds heavier than you were when you reached your goal? Simple. Go back to the regular eating plan until you are at your goal again. Then be careful not to overdo on your free eating days. The key is never to let yourself go over 5 pounds of your goal weight. (Don't worry if from week to week the scale differs by 2 to 3 pounds. Water weight shifts depending upon what you've eaten and, for women, the time of the month.)

It's All in the Thinking

Let's face it. In life we just can't do whatever we want to do. There are certain laws of nature that will stop us cold if we try. So we've got to come to the realization that our bodies are fine-tuned machines. We must feed them with healthy, nutritious food on a regular basis so that they can operate at the maximum. The body will tolerate an occasional indiscretion, but it will not tolerate a continual bombardment of abuse without breaking down (health) and without looking bad (fat). It's that simple.

The good news is, once you become accustomed to eating nutritious foods and learn that you can have your naughty foods on occasion, you will settle in to a happy, healthy lifestyle. After having gotten it off, you will indeed be able to "keep it off."

HEIGHT-WEIGHT CHARTS—YES AND NO!

As you may know by now (if you've read any of my fitness books), I'm not a great advocate of height-weight charts. Becoming obsessed with a number on the scale can be deceiving. Muscle weighs more than fat, but takes up less space, so two people—one with muscle and one without—can be the same height and weight, and one can be two sizes "fatter" than the other! With that aside, height-weight charts can be used as a guide if you take muscle and frame size into account. Here's the chart, but just look at it. Do nothing till you hear from me!

Women*

Height		Small Frame	Medium Frame	Large Frame
(Feet/Inches)				
4	11	98–108	106–118	115–128
5	0	100–110	108–120	117–131
5	1	101–112	110–123	119–134
5	2	103–115	112–126	122–137
5	3	105–118	115–129	125–140
5	4	108–121	118–132	128–144
5	5	111–124	121–135	131–148
5	6	114–127	124–138	134–153
5	7	117–130	127–141	137–156
5	8	120–133	130–144	140–160
5	9	123–136	133–147	142–166
5	10	126–139	136–150	146–167
5	11	129–142	139–153	159–170
6	0	132–145	142–156	162–173
6	1	135–148	145–159	165–176
6	2	138–151	148–162	168–179

*Men add 10 pounds all around.

To use the chart, weigh in the nude and with no shoes. Women who work out with weights and have done so for six months or longer should go by the higher end of the height range. For example, I am medium framed and five feet tall. My ideal weight is 116 to 120 pounds.

But what about your frame? You determine this by measuring the space between your elbow bones, but you need a partner to help you. So get a tape measure and a partner.

With your partner ready with the tape measure, extend your arm and bend your forearm upward at a 90-degree angle. Turn the inside of your wrist toward your body and extend your fingers straight up. Place your thumb and index fingers of your other hand on the bones that protrude on either side of your elbow. Have your partner measure the space between your fingers. (You can't do this yourself because your fingers will probably move and your measurement won't be accurate.)

Height	Space Between Elbow Bones*
4'11"–5'5"	2¼"–2½"
5'6"–5'11"	2⅜"–2⅝"
6'0" and taller	2½"–2¾"

*Men add ¼ inch all around.

After you have gotten the measurement, compare it to those listed in the above chart, which gives the frame determination for a medium framed woman. If your measurement falls within the range of the chart, you are medium framed. If it falls below those given in the chart, you are small framed. If it falls higher, you are large framed.

Now you know your frame and can use the height-weight chart if you wish to do so.

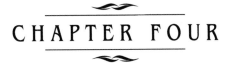

CHAPTER FOUR

COOKING "DELICIOUS" WITHOUT THE FAT

I'm going to help you change your way of thinking when it comes to preparing food, so that eventually you will automatically prepare exciting dishes without fat. Soon you will realize that food is both delicious and appealing—in fact, even more so without that nasty fat we have become so accustomed to using. By the end of this chapter, your mouth will be watering and you'll be eager to try some of the methods mentioned here.

In addition, I'll give you a peek into my refrigerator and food cabinets, so you'll know which manufactured foods I eat on a regular basis as I follow the food plans in this book.

IMPORTANT GENERAL RULES

Some of what you will read in the next paragraph has been discussed in earlier chapters, but not in one place. I summarize it here so that you will have it clearly in your mind—and I'll add some important tips.

Except for the lower-fat exceptions, avoid red meat—and even then, keep it to a bare minimum. When eating poultry, stick to white meat and always remove the skin. In addition, rinse the poultry in cold water while at the same time picking off any fat that may cling to the meat. Do not add any fat of any kind to anything you cook or eat—ever! This means you don't brush the food or the pan lightly with any fatty substance. The only exception to this rule is an occasional nonstick cooking spray, such as Pam, or when I deliberately add canola oil to a meal to fulfill your minimum fat requirement. More about this later.

HOW TO COOK WITHOUT THE FAT

There's a belief that if you can't *taste* the fat, food is not satisfying, substantial, or appealing. In fact, the opposite is true. When you cook without the fat, the food is more satisfying and appealing because fat hides the true flavor of the food. In addition, when you cook without fat, you cook with spices, wines, vinegars, and broths that help to bring out the true flavor of the food.

In the following paragraphs, you'll learn how to broil, sauté, braise, fry, roast, boil, stew, bake, microwave, steam, or pressure-cook food by using a combination of delicious spices, juices, broths, and flavorings. After a few weeks of preparing food this way, your taste buds will change. If you try to go back to your old ways of cooking, you will feel repulsed. Your taste buds will have become accustomed to a more refined palate. In addition, your digestive system will add its confirmation by causing you to feel sluggish and/or slightly nauseated if you switch back to fat-laden, greasy eating.

With this in mind, let's talk about various cooking methods and how you can use them without the fat.

Broiling

When you broil, you cook food by direct heat under or over electric or gas heat—or even between two heated surfaces. Barbecues and rotisseries are also broiling mechanisms; however, the smoke and heat that come from charbroiling create some cancer-causing elements, such as nitrosamine. (If you do barbecue, keep the food as far away from the coals as possible.)

You can use red or white wine as a coating on anything you broil—and I do mean anything! You may already know this, but did you know that you can also use any flavored vinegar, including balsamic, or any juice, such as orange, lemon, tomato, apple, lemon, or lime, to broil foods? For example, if you coat a chicken breast with lemon or lime juice, you actually bring out the full flavor of the chicken. You'll know this is happening because you can smell a delicious aroma after about five minutes of broiling.

I love to broil red peppers, onions, and mushrooms sprinkled with garlic powder, paprika, pepper, and oregano. I don't cut holes in the foil to allow the juice to drip into the pan. I want the juice to remain on the foil so I can scoop it onto the plate with my vegetables when they're done. As this delicious combination cooks, the vegetables yield up a liquid, and the spices seep into that liquid, creating an aromatic juice. The best part is that these vegetables are in the unlimited complex carbohydrate group. If after eating one batch of this broiled mixture I want to make another even bigger batch, I can do so. And it takes only about 7 minutes to do it.

Frying, Sautéing, and Braising

Frying, sautéing, and braising are similar methods of cooking. When you fry food, you brown it in a coating of liquid, traditionally fat. Here, of course, we change the liquid to a spray of vegetable oil or a coating of broth, juice, vinegar, or wine.

When you sauté food, you cook it over high heat in a hot liquid, traditionally fat. Now you will use broth, wine, juice, or vinegar, of course.

Braising is a combination of frying and sautéing. First you fry or brown the food and then you simmer it in a hot liquid in a covered pan.

Replacing fat with the above-mentioned food items will make your fried, braised, or sautéed food taste so much better and will save you hundreds of calories and countless fat grams. For example, instead of sautéing onions in 2 tablespoons of butter, which have 200 calories and 23 grams of fat, you can use a packet of chicken broth that has 10 calories and no fat at all.

The beauty of cooking without fat is that it forces you to become creative. You can pick and choose among the wines, juices, vinegars, and broths and add spices of your choice.

But why bother with all this? With the advent of vegetable cooking spray, which yields almost no fat, and nonstick pans, you can easily fry without the fat. But sooner or later you'll get bored with this low-fat cooking and wax philosophical—and start talking about how life is too short, and it's not worth it (not realizing, of course, that high-fat eating in itself may well ensure that your life *is* short). Using my methods of braising, frying, and sautéing, you'll have the varied taste appeal to keep you on track.

Poaching

You're probably familiar with poaching in the context of eggs, but you can also poach fish or chicken. You can have a succulent, tender meal by placing the fish or chicken in just enough water to cover and coating it with slices of lemon, lime, or orange (after spicing to taste). If you are poaching chicken, it will take about 20 minutes. Fish takes about 5 minutes.

Roasting

When you roast something, you cook it in an oven, over a period of time. Roasting is perhaps the easiest way to cook without fat. Instead of basting the meat with fat drippings, you baste it with broth or juice. The end result is food that is succulent and flavorful.

Let's use chicken or turkey as an example. Remove the skin and baste the meat with your choice of the broth, wine, or juice and, of course, add your spices. When the poultry is cooked, refrigerate the drippings, and after a few hours, remove the fat from the drippings. You can now use the drippings for a gravy base.

If you don't like the idea of skinning a whole chicken or turkey before roasting, you can roast the bird with the skin and remove it later. In this case you won't want to bother using spices and juices for basting. It will be wasted, since all the flavor will go into the skin, which will be removed later. Instead, use the drippings for the basting (so the skin won't burn or char and cause a fire in your oven) and then remove the bird from the oven about 10 to 15 minutes before it is done. Now you can remove the skin. Put the poultry back in the oven and use the basting methods mentioned above after adding spices. Cook until done (10 to 15 minutes). The flavors of the basting and spices will seep into the chicken or turkey.

Boiling and Stewing

Boiling is cooking in water that is 212°F. or hotter, or until the water bubbles, and then continuing to cook with the bubbles until the food is done. Stewing is cooking over low heat, after the food has boiled.

You can boil potatoes with the skins on or off and season them after they are done. If you're boiling new potatoes, you will be able to leave the skins on. Corn on the cob is another excellent choice for boiling. Carrots, broccoli, and cauliflower—and any vegetable, for that matter—can also be boiled, but they take a little longer, and you lose some of the vitamins and minerals into the water. I'd rather use the microwave or the pressure cooker for them, or even the steamer.

Good old-fashioned boiling and then simmering (a form of stewing) is my favorite way to make chicken soup. I throw in the pot two skinned chicken breasts, a packet of supermarket "soup greens" (turnips, fresh parsley, carrots, onions, etc.), a few extra onions and carrots, and some seasonings and let it come to a boil. Then I reduce the heat to a simmer and go about my business. In about 20 minutes the flavor of the cooking soup calls me and I look in on it. In another 15 to 25 minutes, the soup is ready. Now all I do is add instant rice and wait about 5 minutes. Wow, what a soup.

Even though a pressure cooker is much faster for stewing, I sometimes toss a bunch of vegetables into a pot with a soup bone (the butcher will give you one for free), and let it "stew" for an hour or more.

Microwaving

The microwave oven is the only cooking method that, instead of cooking food from the outside in, cooks food from the inside out! I must admit that I fought the idea of microwaving until about two years ago. Now I ask myself, "Where have I been all my life?" For certain foods and certain occasions, the microwave is a gift from God. I use it to make my fish stews (recipes in Chapter 7) and to bake a whole fresh cauliflower (wrapped in microwave plastic wrap and cooked on high for 7 minutes). Once in a while I cut up a bunch of vegetables, put them in a microwave dish, add spices, and cook them on high for about 10 minutes.

I also use the microwave to bake potatoes (about 6 minutes on high), sweet potatoes (about 7 minutes on high), or yams (about 8 minutes on high). The microwave is also great for making corn on the cob (without removing the husks, for about 10 minutes).

I don't like the microwave oven for chicken or beef (I rarely eat beef), but I love it for fish! It takes only about 2 minutes to cook 4 to 6 ounces of fish. After spicing the fish, I put it into a microwave dish and add a little water to the bottom of the dish so the fish comes out moist and steamy.

Pressure Cooking

Pressure-cooked food is cooked at extremely high temperatures under the pressure created by the cooker mechanism. The pressure cooker was the microwave of the fifties! To this day, l remember the *tcc tccc tchh* rocking sound of the pressure cooker that held a hearty stew my mother was cooking for dinner.

These days, hardly anyone uses a pressure cooker. I often wonder why, but I think it was replaced by the microwave. This should not be—the pressure cooker offers an entirely different food result. The food comes out tasting like it's been stewed or boiled, whereas the microwave yields a more baked or broiled effect.

When you pressure-cook, you get a time bomb of flavor in a matter of minutes. You can stew vegetables—with or without poultry, fish, or meat, in combination with various spices—experimenting to please your inclination. You can discover for yourself a variety of virtually fat-free pressure-cooked combinations. (Be sure to write to me with some of your discoveries so that I can use them too, and maybe they'll be included in the *Joyce Vedral Newsletter*; see page 346.)

Steaming

Steamed food is cooked by boiling water so that steam surrounds the food and eventually cooks it. Because the food never comes into direct contact with the cooking source (water, coals, coils), steaming is one of the purest ways of cooking. For example, if you steam rather than boil vegetables, you won't lose any of the vitamin content. Also, you can get the vegetables to cook to just the right consistency—not too soft, not too hard, and not too charred.

You can purchase a vegetable steamer in any department store (Black and Decker's Handy Steamer is an excellent choice) and steam broccoli, cauliflower, carrots, squash, onions, and so on. You can also steam rice and a variety of other items.

Baking

When you bake something, you cook it in an oven in temperatures ranging from 150 to 500°F. Baking is associated with fattening items such as cakes, cookies, pies, muffins, and croissants.

There was once a time when dieters had to give up baked goods completely because baking always meant fat. Today, as you well know, you can purchase a variety of nonfat baked goods. But many of these food items are high in sugar! So how can you bake your own foods without the fat? You can use many substitutes; these will be explained as you read the rest of this chapter. No longer will you have to use fatty egg yolks, butter, margarine, or oil in your baking. You'll be able to bake breads, cakes, and cookies without the fat! And you can use juice concentrate in place of sugar. I'll give you some simple recipes for baked goods in Chapter 8, but later in this chapter I'll give you some general rules that you can apply to your own baking.

A FEW HANDY COOKING ITEMS

Aside from the three cooking items mentioned above—the pressure cooker, the microwave oven, and the steamer—there are two more cooking items you should have.

First, you'll need an assortment of nonstick cookware: frying pan, muffin pan, cookie sheet, and square, rectangular, and/or loaf pans. You can purchase nonstick cookware in any major department store. It will make your frying and baking life much easier, and will keep your need to use vegetable oil spray to a minimum.

Second, a food processor. You can use it to combine vegetables into a thick liquid, which can then be used as a base for stews, gravies, soups—you name it! This machine can chip, puree, slice, shred, blend, and knead, even whip egg whites. An excellent brand is Cuisinart.

HERBS AND SPICES TO MAKE YOU FORGET ABOUT FAT

Herbs and spices can make the difference between hating the food on a low-fat eating plan and loving it. If it were not for spices, I think I would have no choice but to be fat! Spices can make any food appealing to the taste.

There are spices that will complement any food you cook, whether broiled, braised, boiled, poached, microwaved, pressure-cooked, or steamed. Use the following as a guideline, and then experiment until you find the particular combinations that work for you. (Note that the "powders" are not "salts." That's very important! If you buy the salt instead of the powder, you'll load your food with unnecessary sodium.)

Poultry: Basil, bay leaf, chervil, chili powder, chives, cumin, curry, dill, garlic powder, ginger, marjoram, onion powder, oregano, mustard powder, mustard seed, paprika, parsley, pepper, rosemary, saffron, sage, tarragon, thyme.

Fish: Basil, bay leaf, celery seed, chervil, chili powder, coriander, curry, dill, fennel, garlic powder, onion powder, oregano, pepper, paprika, parsley, rosemary, saffron, tarragon.

Meats (for later, when you've reached your goal): Basil, bay leaf, chili powder, cloves, coriander, cumin, curry, fennel, garlic powder, ginger, marjoram, mint, mustard powder, mustard seed, onion powder, oregano, pepper, rosemary, savory, thyme.

Soups and Vegetables: Allspice, basil, bay leaf, capers, celery seed, chives, cloves, coriander, dill, fennel, ginger, horseradish, mace, marjoram, mustard, mustard seed, onion powder, parsley, oregano, pepper, rosemary, saffron, savory, sesame seed, sage, tarragon, thyme.

Salt Substitutes: There are about 500 milligrams of salt in ¼ teaspoon of salt, so you may be able to well afford the optional salt offerings in the recipes. However, if you wish to substitute for salt (and avoid the chemical-laden substitutes), use a combination of celery seed, garlic powder, lemon juice, onion powder, and Tabasco sauce. You may also opt for the light salt, which has about 275 milligrams of sodium per ¼ teaspoon, or Papa Dash's Lite Salt, which has only 90 milligrams of sodium per ¼ teaspoon.

You can experiment with these herbs and spices and see which ones appeal to your taste buds. You can also dare to combine them in any way your mood leads you. For example, if you're cooking some fish in the microwave, put the fish in a microwave dish, then add any combination of spices listed for fish.

You can also slice up some tomatoes, onions, mushrooms, or squash, add it to the fish mixture with about 1½ cups water, and cook it for 15 minutes on high. Your end result will be a sort of fish chowder, to which you can add some instant rice. If you wait 5 minutes after adding the rice, you'll have a huge bowl of hearty fish-rice soup and you'll be able to eat the whole thing without guilt. The only fat in the dish is the fat in your low-fat fish. If you don't like a lot of protein, you can put the bare minimum of fish—4 ounces, or even less—in the pot and you'll still get that delicious fish flavor.

When I'm broiling chicken, I remove the skin and then sprinkle both sides with paprika, garlic powder, oregano, and basil. Or, after removing the skin, I sprinkle the chicken with lemon juice, rosemary, sage, and thyme. If I'm broiling fish, I may sprinkle it with dill, celery seed, and tarragon one day, and coriander, curry, and fennel the next.

If I'm sautéing vegetables in a thin layer of water, I may add chives, dill, onion powder, and pepper. Sometimes I go wild and put in nearly every spice on the list. You can really have fun experimenting with spices. You can really change the flavor of vegetables if you add appropriate spices. It's one way to "get them down" if you don't particularly like vegetables. A little parsley, dill, coriander, or dry mustard can make you wonder if your steamed broccoli is broccoli at all!

When preparing a delicious soup once again, you can experiment but keep in mind what's in the soup. For example, if it's chicken soup, you'll want to stick to the chicken spices that coincide with the vegetable spices. But what if you want to ignore the lists and just use herbs and spices anywhere, any time, at your own whim? Of course, do it. There's no law that says you can't use them; it's just that cooks have found these herbs and spices to go best with these foods. You may disagree and who knows, you may invent some new dishes.

MAKING RICE, POTATOES, OR PASTA MORE INTERESTING

Try cooking rice (and any vegetable, for that matter) in half water and half vegetable or tomato juice with chopped onions and spices. If you don't mind sweet rice, you can use other juices, such as orange, apple, or pineapple.

Mash your potatoes without fat. Use water and skim milk and add spices. I add a little salt, pepper, and paprika; when I'm in the mood, I add a sprinkle of Butter Buds.

You can have a semblance of French-fried potatoes in sliced form. Slice the potatoes thinly and "fry" them in a nonstick pan with paprika, lemon juice, salt, and pepper; or cut a new potato into eight parts and sprinkle with these seasonings, then place in a microwave on high for 7 minutes.

Tomato sauce for pasta doesn't have to contain any fat. You can flavor canned tomatoes with garlic powder and either Italian seasoning or oregano and bay leaves. You can also opt to use tomato paste and add water and spices of your choice. Another way to go is to simply sauté 3 chopped fresh tomatoes in a cup of red wine and oregano, garlic powder, and any other spices you choose. After 15 minutes, mix this into your pasta and you have a scrumptious meal.

You can make a white sauce for your pasta by using nonfat milk and cornstarch and any combination of spices.

MAKING SANDWICHES INTERESTING WITHOUT FAT

You can learn to develop a taste for mustard instead of mayonnaise. I've done it and now I can't stand the idea of mayonnaise on anything except tomato and lettuce sandwiches on whole wheat toast—and then I'm happy with the nonfat mayonnaise.

Chicken or turkey breast sandwiches are quite delicious with regular brown or yellow mustard if you add tomatoes and lettuce for juice and flavor. Or, use red-hot sauce or salsa—mild, medium, or hot. You could also add sliced cucumbers, pickled red peppers or pimientos, or sliced pickles to make the sandwich juicy.

Another approach is to make a sandwich spread by adding a variety of spices to nonfat mayonnaise. For example, you can add chili powder or crushed red pepper to the mayonnaise.

Broiled eggplant, tomatoes, and onions can make quite a delicious sandwich. When I'm really hungry and I've used up my protein allotment, I'll make such a concoction and put it on two slices of nonfat whole wheat bread. It's so delicious that I usually have two, for the price of a limited complex carbohydrate allotment. If I've used up that allotment, I'll just eat the mix without the bread, putting it on lettuce if I want the feel of a sandwich.

You can make your tuna-in-water sandwiches more interesting by chopping some cucumbers into the mix. Add onions and other vegetables, depending upon your mood. You can even add spices and experiment with different flavored vinegars. Of course, there is always nonfat mayonnaise.

Marinated cucumber sandwiches are also delicious. I like to slice and soak a cucumber overnight in red wine and spices with a little vinegar added. Then I use the mix for two or three sandwiches during the course of the day, adding lettuce to hold some of the juice.

You can always make your sandwiches more appealing by daring to do the unusual. Who is stopping you from thinly slicing red peppers, cucumbers, radishes, red onions, and carrots and adding them to your sandwich? Or even better, making a sandwich out of some such combination? Let's not forget that you can also microwave the vegetables for 7 minutes and then stuff them into a whole wheat pita bread.

EXCITING NONFAT SALADS AND DRESSINGS

Some days I have at least three huge salads. When I'm lazy, I just throw some romaine lettuce in a bowl with tomatoes, garlic, wine vinegar, and a little salt. When I'm more patient, I'll cut up some cucumbers, onions, red peppers, and maybe some radishes and carrots, and add them to the mix. I don't always use romaine lettuce. I buy all different kinds of lettuce and mix them together. I can eat as many salads as I please in a given day without breaking my diet.

Dressing up the Salad

Why bother to make the salad interesting? Because if you don't, when you go to your refrigerator and think of making a salad, you'll close the door and walk away in defeat. "Eh, I'd rather go hungry," you'll say. Then a few minutes later, when your daughter is munching on her potato chips (she gets them whether you like it or not), and she goes to answer a phone call, leaving the chips behind, you steal one, then two, then half the bag!

Here are some general rules for making salads.

1. Use a variety of lettuces. Go to your produce department and ask the names of various kinds of lettuce and try them.

2. Add various vegetables to your lettuce base: strips of red and/or green pepper, rings of red onions, chopped white onions, sliced or diced cucumbers, or kirby (small pickling) cucumbers, pickles, hot peppers, roasted peppers, mushrooms, radishes, or bits of broccoli. Of course, you're not going to throw all of the above into a salad (but then you may), but experiment and find the combinations that make you happy.

3. Make your own roasted red peppers by slicing up a few and broiling them on a piece of foil for 20 minutes. They're delicious even if unevenly cooked and partially burned. You can cut them up and mix them into the salad.

4. Toss some sauerkraut into the salad.

5. Add a tablespoon of chick-peas or kidney beans, flavored bread crumbs, or chopped beets.

6. Add ½ cup of cooked tricolor pasta.

7. Make your own nonfat "croutons" by flavoring some peas as you will and broiling them for 15 minutes. Sprinkle the peas on the top of the salad.

Note: Chick-peas, kidney beans, pasta, bread crumbs, and peas are not allowed in unlimited amounts, but if you use a very small amount—say, 1 or 2 tablespoons—you can have them for free—no more than once a day.

Dressing up the Dressing

A shake or two of salt and/or some chosen spices, sprinkled with a little water, may be all you need for a burst of flavor, depending upon the combination of vegetables in the salad. Or, you can use lemon or lime juice or any flavored vinegar as a base for your salad dressing and then add the spices of your choice. You can also crush some fresh garlic and mix it into the salad.

Sometimes I just use a few tablespoons of mild salsa as my salad dressing, along with some wine or rice vinegar, or I make a creamy type dressing by using either nonfat plain yogurt, buttermilk, or sour cream, adding spices or flavored vinegar to fit my mood. Other times I sprinkle my salad with mustard powder and water and add a few spices.

Use a food processor to make a salad dressing by pureeing some vegetables, such as tomatoes, carrots, onions, and red peppers, mixed with a little water and/or lemon or lime juice or flavored vinegar along with some spices.

You can always use the nonfat dressings, but some of them are even higher in calories, spoon for spoon, than the ones that contain fat. Try to avoid any nonfat salad dressing that is more than 5 calories per serving.

GENERAL TRICKS TO GET THE FAT OUT

There are literally hundreds of books that give excellent tips for getting the fat out of your food, many of them so time-consuming that it depresses me just to think of trying them. I'm going to give you what I consider to be the most useful and realistic tips—ones that I use myself on a regular basis. Some of them may seem to be common sense, though they were not always so to me. Others may seem to be very "uncommon" sense, in fact hardly believable. For the obvious, I apologize; for the not so believable, I ask you to try them!

1. Skim the fat from soup. Whenever you make soup with a fat-containing food item, after cooking, refrigerate the soup until the fat solidifies, then skim all the fat from the top. The fat on canned soups (before cooking) will already be on the top. You can immediately skim it off and you'll be reducing the stated fat content a great deal. (I don't want you to now think this is license to purchase soups with high fat contents and then skim the fat and think, "Okay, now I have no fat grams." You must count the fat grams on the label anyway, but skim the fat and know you are getting a bonus of less fat than you've accounted for.)

2. Use thickeners instead of fat for a gravy base. Instead of using the fat drippings from meat, defat the drippings by cooking and removing the fat, and add to the drippings 2 table-spoons of either barley flour, arrowroot, cornmeal, or corn-starch. Flavor to taste. (You can use low-sodium soy sauce as a salt substitute if you choose.) Amazingly, you will have a fat-less gravy.

3. If you crave nuts, eat chestnuts or baked oatmeal instead. Chestnuts are about 60 calories an ounce, and they have just over a half a gram of fat, whereas peanuts have about 180 calories and 14 grams of fat! Another idea is to take some oatmeal (the instant won't work; use the old-fashioned kind), add some cinnamon or nutmeg and maybe some artificial sweet-ener, and spread it on an aluminum foil–lined broiler pan and broil for about 10 minutes. Turn the oats about every 3 minutes. When done, they will be crunchy, like nuts.

4. Bake apples, bananas, or oranges instead of eating fat-laden candy. You can bake up a batch of apples, oranges, or bananas, or a combination, spicing them according to your taste. When I bake apples, I remove the core and fill it with a few raisins, some cinnamon, and a little artificial sweetener. For bananas, I use white wine, nutmeg, and a little artificial sweet-ener. For oranges, I use mint and artificial sweetener. I bake them for anywhere from 10 to 20 minutes.

You can sweeten the fruit (or any other food item, for that matter) with pure, concentrated fruit juice instead of sugar or other sweet substances, or you can make up a liqueur-tasting combination such as apple juice concentrate and vanilla and almond extract (to taste like Amaretto), or orange juice con-centrate and vanilla extract (to taste like Grand Marnier), or apple juice concentrate, rum, and coconut extract to taste like a piña colada.

5. Use evaporated milk instead of whipped cream. You can get a substance that is much like whipped cream by whipping up some cold evaporated milk (make sure the bowl is refrigerated for at least an hour before you do the whipping). Whip until the milk is thick enough to look like whipped cream.

6. Use pureed vegetables or beans instead of fatty meats or roux. You can thicken a soup or stew with pureed vegetables or beans (see the unlimited and limited complex carbohydrates lists on pages 66 and 67 and pages 68 and 69) instead of using fatty meats or roux (a mixture of butter and flour commonly used to thicken soups). You'll need a food processor for this. Simply remove half of the vegetables cooking in the soup, puree them in the food processor, and then return them to the soup mixture.

7. Use nonfat yogurt or cottage cheese for sour cream. Of course, you can always simply use nonfat sour cream. But I can't do that. For some reason, I want to eat the whole container of sour cream and then the calories add up. So I have to stick to the nonfat yogurt or cottage cheese, where 2 tablespoons are not a temptation.

8. Put salsa on baked potatoes instead of butter or sour cream. If you change your thinking about what does and does not go on potatoes, you may decide to try salsa. I use either mild or medium salsa; the salsa is only about 10 calories a serving, so even if I go to town and use three or four servings, what damage am I really doing?

9. Use applesauce to replace fat in any recipe. Yes. You heard right. Measure for measure, applesauce can take the place of fat in any recipe, as long as the flavors blend. Apple is a neutral flavor so it doesn't dominate the taste of most dishes. For example, if the recipe calls for 1 tablespoon of fat, replace it for 1 tablespoon of applesauce and you'll have a delicious result, without the fat.

10. Use egg whites for egg yolks. When a recipe calls for whole eggs, simply leave out the yolks and double the whites. For example, if a recipe calls for two eggs, use four whites. There are about 5 grams of fat in each egg yolk, whereas there is no fat in egg whites. And as you know, the fat in egg yolks is also the artery-clogging fat that raises bad cholesterol levels! (Or sidestep this by using a commercial egg-replacement product, such as Egg Beaters. As a general rule, I prefer using egg whites.) Note: Most doctors agree that it is okay to eat up to three egg yolks per week.

11. Use lactose-reduced or lactose-free skim milk instead of 1 percent milk—and never use nondairy creamers. One percent milk has about 100 calories a glass and 2.6 grams of fat, but skim milk has 86 calories a glass and no fat. You'd be surprised how much fat you can save by just this little sacrifice—using skim milk instead of 1% milk. And you'll be amazed how once you get used to it, you won't even miss that fat.

Up until now I resented using skim milk because I didn't think it made my coffee light enough. But I discovered that the lactose-free skim milk makes my coffee lighter than regular skim milk. In other words, when I use lactose-free skim milk, it feels as if I'm using at least 1% milk. (If I use 1% lactose-free milk, it feels as if I'm using 2% milk.) This has been a great discovery for me, because now I can enjoy my coffee with no fat at all. And, there's a bonus: lactose-reduced and lactose-free milk does not spoil for six weeks or more! Why does this make me so happy? I can buy loads of it, and I find that I don't run out of milk as often.

Nondairy creamers (made from tropical oils) used to be a lifesaver for those who were lactose intolerant, but now that we have lactose-reduced and lactose-free milk, they have outgrown their use. They are and always were more fattening than full-fat milk! A mere teaspoon of nondairy creamer has 10 calories and a whopping gram of fat! Most people use 2 to 3 teaspoons—or more—in a cup of coffee. In the course of a day you can consume 10 grams of fat in just creamer alone. What a waste of your fat allotment.

12. Put a piece of tape over your mouth when you're cooking. I'm not kidding! If you're like me, when you're cooking one spoon goes in the mouth after each stir! In order to retrain yourself not to taste while cooking, put tape over your mouth for one week when cooking. After that you'll be aware of your tasting, and perhaps be able to get it under control. Having done this, mysteriously, you'll find yourself losing weight much faster than before.

IF YOU LOOK IN MY FOOD CABINETS OR REFRIGERATOR, YOU'LL FIND . . .

The following is a list of my favorite food staples that can be purchased at any supermarket or food store. At any given time, you will find a combination of these specific foods in my home. Of course, I don't want you to feel in any way limited to the foods or brands I mention, but I do want you to know what I really eat, other than the foods outlined in Chapter 3.

Pasta and No-Egg Noodles

De Boles American (Jerusalem) Artichoke Natural Gourmet Pasta, Whole Wheat Pasta, Spaghetti-Style Pasta
Contadina Protein-Enriched Pasta
Ronzoni Orzo
No Yolks Cholesterol-Free Egg Noodle Substitute
Pennsylvania Dutch Yolk-Free Ribbons (egg noodle substitute)

Sauces

Classico Mushrooms and Ripe Olives Sauce, Spicy Red Pepper Sauce, Tomato and Basil Sauce
Aunt Millie's Italian-Style Spaghetti Sauce (flavored with meat, marinara)

Healthy Choice Garlic and Herbs Pasta Sauce (and other flavors)
Redpack Whole Tomatoes, Sliced Tomatoes, Tomato Paste
Pope Whole Tomatoes, Crushed Tomatoes, Tomato Paste
Ragu Fino Italian Brand Zesty Tomato Sauce
Campbell's Low-Sodium V-8 Juice (I heat it up and use it as a sauce for pasta)

Rice

Uncle Ben's Natural Whole-Grain Instant Brown Rice
Minute Original Instant Enriched White Rice
Panella Arroz

Barley

Mother's Quick Cooking Barley

Bread and English Muffins

Arnold's Bakery Light Golden Wheat
Roman Meal 100% Whole Wheat Bread
Wonder Lite, Reduced Calorie, and Fat-Free Breads (any whole-grain)
Beefsteak Light Soft Rye
Mr. Pita 100% Whole Wheat Pocket Pita
Toufayan Pita (whole wheat)
Thomas's English Muffins (Oat Bran, Regular, or any variety)

Cereals

Pritikin Multigrain Hot Cereal, Apple Spice Hot Cereal
H.O. Old-Fashioned Oats, 100% Whole-Grain Oats
Quaker Instant Oatmeal, Apples & Cinnamon (or any other flavor)

Health Valley Bran Cereal
Nabisco Shredded Wheat
Quaker Puffed Wheat or Puffed Rice
General Mills Fiber One

Milk

Lactaid Lactose-Reduced 1% or Skim Milk
Lactaid Lactose-Free 1% or Skim Milk
Carnation Evaporated Low-fat Milk
Alba Nonfat Evaporated Milk

Ice Cream and Frozen Yogurt

Borden's Fat-Free Ice Cream
Dryer's (Edy's) Fat-Free Ice Cream
Yoplait Fat-Free Yogurt
Breyer's Fat-Free Yogurt

Other Dairy Items

Butter Buds (sprinkle and mix to liquid)
Kraft Free Mayonnaise and Miracle Whip
Weight Watcher's Fat-Free Mayonnaise
Pam or Wesson Spray
Land O' Lakes or Light & Lively Fat-Free Sour Cream and
    Cottage Cheese
Dannon or Yoplait Plain Nonfat Yogurt
Polly-O Free Fat-Free Mozzarella
Alpine Lace Fat-Free American or Cheddar Cheese
Healthy Choice Nonfat American or Cheddar Cheese

(*Note:* I rarely keep ice cream, sour cream, or cheese—too tempting—but once in a while for certain occasions I dare to include these foods.)

Vinegar

Regina Red Wine Vinegar with Garlic

Soups and Broth

Campbell's Healthy Request Hearty Chicken Rice Soup (try
    others but watch the label for calories and fat grams)
Pritikin Hearty Vegetable, Pasta, Minestrone Soup
Healthy Choice Chicken with Rice Soup
Health Valley Fat-Free Soup, 14 Garden Vegetables
Progresso Healthy Classics (especially Chicken Noodle)
Progresso Soups (especially Hearty Chicken)
Herb-Ox Instant Broth and Seasoning, Chicken, Beef
Herb-Ox Instant Broth and Seasoning, Very Low Sodium
    Chicken, Beef
Campbell's Healthy Request Fat-Free Chicken Broth
Mother's Low-Calorie Borscht (that's the Russian in me)

Fish

Bumble Bee Solid White, Chunk White, Light Tuna in Water
Starkist Solid White, Chunk White, Light Tuna in Water

Chicken and Turkey

Healthy Choice Lite Sliced or Whole Chicken or Turkey
    Breast

Pickles, Hot Peppers, Roasted Peppers, Salsa

Ba-Tempte Kosher Dills
Ba-Tempte Half Sour Pickles
Featherweight Whole Dill Pickles
B & G Hot Red Cherry Peppers
Mancini Roasted Peppers
Enrique Salsa Piquante

Cookies, Cakes, Crackers, Frozen Desserts

SnackWell's Fat-Free Cinnamon Graham Snacks
Nabisco Fat-Free Saltine Crackers
Devonshire Plain Melba Rounds
Weight Watcher's Cakes and Brownies (be aware of fat
   grams and calories)
Good Humor Sugar-Free Popsicles (Ice-Pops)

Pretzels, Popcorn, Raisins

Eagle Pretzels, Sourdough Hard Bavarian, Fat-Free
Rold Gold, Baked Fat-Free Pretzels (any variety)
Mr. Salty Pretzel Sticks
Orville Redenbacher's Smart Pop Low-Fat Microwave Popcorn
Sunmaid California Sun-Dried Raisins

Jell-O and Canned Fruit

Jell-O Fat-Free Jell-O (not the puddings—they add up to too
    many calories)
Libby's Natural Lite Fruit Cocktail, Pears, Peaches
Diet Delight Fruit Cocktail, Pears, Peaches

Hot Chocolate and Teas

Swiss Miss Sugar-Free Hot Chocolate
Swiss Miss Fat-Free Hot Chocolate
Carnation Sugar-Free Hot Chocolate
Celestial Seasonings Chamomile Tea and other flavors

Condiments

Enrico's Catsup
Featherweight Unsalted Prepared Mustard
Kikkoman, Westbrae Mild Soy Sauce
Tabasco sauce
Goya Sazón (seasoning)

Salad Dressing

Pritikin Garlic and Herb Dressing, French, Vinaigrette,
    Ranch, Sweet and Spicy, Italian

CHAPTER FIVE

BREAKFAST MENUS FOR A MONTH

Breakfast is said to be the most important meal of the day. It's the meal that literally "breaks your fast," the fast that even the most constant eaters engage in during sleep.

Why should you eat breakfast, especially if you say, "I'm not hungry in the morning"? Perhaps you get up at six or seven o'clock in the morning to go to work, grabbing only a quick cup of coffee, and you don't eat until about noon. You've been up five or six hours and you haven't eaten a thing—and what's more, you don't care! Let me motivate you to change your ways. If you want to lose weight, you'll eat something in the morning. It doesn't have to be a lot, but something.

If you deprive your body of food—any time between three and five hours—your metabolism dramatically slows down to cope with what it perceives as a threat to its well-being. In short, your body says to itself, "There may be a famine coming up. I'd better conserve energy to stay alive." You experience this metabolic slowdown as a slight sensation of tiredness. But what has really happened is that your body is now burning fewer calories than it would have burned doing the same task. On the other hand, had you had a light breakfast, even a slice or two of whole wheat bread, your body would have done the opposite—it would have energized and gone into high gear, kicking up your metabolism to burn the fuel you just put into it.

In addition, when you don't eat breakfast you don't function at optimum capacity. When you deprive your body of food all morning, you're actually running on limited mental and physical capacity—and you're doing yourself and your boss (if you're working) a tremendous disservice.

Just think. You could have eaten breakfast, felt better, been less grouchy, functioned more efficiently, and lost more weight in the bargain. But what did you do? You told yourself, secretly, "I'll save my food for later—why waste it now. I'm not really hungry and I'm in a hurry, anyway." In the back of your mind you believed that you would lose more weight this way—but now you know better, so dare to change your ways. Remember, the wise man said, "The definition of insanity is to keep doing the same thing, and expect something different to happen." Hello!

So let's agree that even if you're not really hungry, you'll eat something in the morning. It doesn't have to be an elaborate meal. And if you're in a hurry, you can choose one of the quickie breakfasts in this chapter—or you can simply eat two slices of 45-calorie whole wheat bread on the run. That's much better than nothing, and it will keep your metabolism and mental and physical energy up.

In the following pages, you will find thirty-one breakfast menus and seven ultra-quickie breakfasts. The first ten menus are quickie meals and the next seven are ultra-quickie (so quick that I'm not even counting them as part of the thirty-one breakfasts). The next twenty-one take more time, but can be prepared in advance and used as quickies, especially the muffins. (I bake two dozen at a time and freeze them.)

UNDERSTANDING THE NUTRITIONAL INFORMATION

Following each recipe are one or more nutritional analyses listing the calorie content plus protein, fat, sodium, and carbohydrate found in the food. The calculations are *per serving* unless otherwise indicated. For example, in a recipe serving four persons, the analysis will be for one serving. For a recipe yielding six pancakes, three pancakes constituting a serving, the analysis will be for three pancakes.

You will note that when a fruit or a vegetable is added as a side dish, the calculations are shown separately—one analysis for the main dish and one for the side dish—so that you have detailed information on the food values of the specific foods you are eating. Also, if you are using the recipes to make up your own meal plans, you might want to eliminate or substitute the side dish.

Protein and fat measures are shown in grams (g); sodium and carbohydrate contents are given in milligrams (mg). Refer to Chapter 3 for guidelines on using these figures. Bear in mind, however, that the meal plans in Chapter 9 count everything for you—these analyses are for your information in case you want to make your own daily meal plans.

When an alternative ingredient appears in parentheses, this means the substitute has not been included in the analysis. For example, "1 teaspoon garlic powder (or salt)" means that the analysis includes garlic powder but not salt (which would yield a higher sodium content).

When recipes include wheat germ or canola oil, the analysis for these items is usually kept separate. I've added these items in the recipe to meet the fat requirements in the meal plans, but if you are developing your own meal plans, you might want to omit these items and obtain your fat minimum in another way. In the rare cases when it is included in the recipe, it is because I feel it is absolutely necessary to the taste of the recipe.

A NOTE ABOUT THE RECIPES

Where nonstick cookware is involved, it is assumed that you have lightly coated the cookware with a vegetable oil cooking spray, like Pam.

When 1 percent dairy products are used, or regular granola, feel free to substitute nonfat products. I use the 1 percent items when I feel you need that bit of fat to fulfill a healthy daily fat requirement. (The minimum fat you should get is 10 percent of total caloric intake.)

Feel free to substitute the fruit or vegetable on the side with any other fruit or vegetable, or eliminate the item at the meal and eat it any other time of the day. Also feel free to cut the serving size if you feel it is too much for you.

Fruits and vegetables in the ingredients lists are medium size unless otherwise indicated. Herbs and spices are dried unless fresh is indicated.

When making muffins, follow the directions for baking time; however, don't completely rely on that figure. Always put a toothpick into the center of the muffin to see if it comes out without crumbs adhering to it. If it does, it's done. If crumbs adhere, it indicates the muffin is damp inside and needs a few more minutes' cooking time.

QUICKIE BREAKFASTS

1. Bagel and Lox Without the Lox—and with Half a Grapefruit

Serves 1

1 tablespoon low-fat cream cheese
½ bagel, toasted or not, your choice
½ tomato, sliced
½ pickle, sliced
2 onion slices, preferably Spanish onion
½ grapefruit

1. Spread cream cheese over bagel half.
2. Add tomato slices, pickle, and onion on top. It should be piled high. You should have to crank your mouth open to get it in. In fact, you can use a whole bagel and make it a sandwich.
3. Serve with ½ grapefruit.

Bagel
Calories: 102
Protein: 6 g
Fat: 3.4 g
Sodium: 745 mg
Cholesterol: 3 mg

Grapefruit
Calories: 32
Protein: 0.6 g
Fat: 0
Sodium: 1 mg
Cholesterol: 0

2. Bagel and Cream Cheese Sweet Peach Sit-Ups

Serves 1

½ bagel
1 peach, halved and cut into thin slices
1 tablespoon 1% cream cheese
2 teaspoons strawberry jam

1. Toast the bagel.
2. While bagel is toasting, cut peach into thin strips.
3. Spread cream cheese on bagel. Add strawberry jam. Top with thin peach strips.
4. Serve with remaining peach strips on the side.

Calories: 182
Protein: 7.8 g
Fat: 3.6 g
Sodium: 258 mg
Cholesterol: 3 mg

3. Banana-Boat Beauty Queen

Serves 1

1 banana
½ cup nonfat cottage cheese
⅛ teaspoon wheat germ
Sprinkle of cinnamon
Sprinkle of artificial sweetener
2 slices whole wheat toast

1. Split the banana.
2. Arrange cottage cheese in the split.
3. Sprinkle with wheat germ, cinnamon, and sweetener.
4. Serve with whole wheat toast on the side.

Banana Boat
Calories: 237
Protein: 21 g
Fat: 1.3 g
Sodium: 17 mg
Cholesterol: 8 mg

Whole Wheat Toast*
Calories: 112
Protein: 4.8 g
Fat: 1.4 g
Sodium: 242 mg
Cholesterol: 1 mg

4. Three Little Bears on-the-Run Porridge with Pear

Serves 1

1 teaspoon wheat germ
1 35-gram packet instant cinnamon-apple oatmeal
2 tablespoons raisins
⅛ teaspoon nutmeg
⅛ teaspoon cinnamon
⅛ teaspoon almond extract
½ cup boiling water
1 pear, cut into wedges

1. In a medium bowl, combine wheat germ, oatmeal, raisins, nutmeg, and cinnamon. Mix thoroughly.
2. Add almond extract and boiling water and mix thoroughly.
3. Pour into a bowl and sprinkle with an extra dash of cinnamon.
4. Serve with pear wedges on the side.

*You may find whole wheat bread with only 45 calories per slice—but if not, 56 is fine.

Porridge
Calories: 227
Protein: 10 g
Fat: 4.3 g
Sodium: 3 mg
Cholesterol: 0

Pears
Calories: 118
Protein: 0.8 g
Fat: 0.8 g
Sodium: 0
Cholesterol: 0

5. Hearty Oatmeal and Mango Day Starter

Serves 1

½ cup water
½ cup old-fashioned oats
Sprinkle of salt (optional)
1 small mango, cut into slices
Sprinkle of cinnamon (or Tabasco sauce)
Sprinkle of sugar (or artificial sweetener)

1. Bring water to a boil in small saucepan.
2. Add oats and salt. Cook for 2 minutes over high heat.
3. Lower heat, cover, and cook for 1 more minute.
4. Arrange mango slices on a plate. Sprinkle oatmeal with cinnamon and sugar or sweetener or, if you prefer, Tabasco sauce. Serve with piping hot oatmeal.

Note: I love oatmeal and live on it in the morning. It is the most energy-supplying low-fat food I know. I use Tabasco sauce to give it some zing.

Oatmeal
Calories: 163
Protein: 6.8 g
Fat: 2.7 g
Sodium: 2 mg
Cholesterol: 0

Mango Slices
Calories: 131
Protein: 1 g
Fat: 0.6 g
Sodium: 4 mg
Cholesterol: 0

6. Cold Cereal Quickie with Strawberries

Serves 1

1 cup puffed wheat cereal
¾ cup 1% milk
3 large strawberries, sliced

1. Place cereal in a bowl.
2. Pour on milk.
3. Add sliced strawberries.

Note: You may use any other low-fat cold cereal, such as Fiber One.

Calories: 200
Protein: 11 g
Fat: 3.5 g
Sodium: 96 mg
Cholesterol: 4 mg

7. English Muffin Motivation with Grapes

Serves 1

½ whole wheat English muffin
½ tomato, cut into 4 slices
1 slice nonfat American cheese
Sprinkle of salt (or onion powder)
Sprinkle of dill
Small bunch of grapes (about 20)

1. Cover English muffin with 2 tomato slices.
2. Place American cheese on top of tomatoes.
3. Sprinkle with salt or onion powder and dill.
4. Place 2 more tomato slices over cheese and again sprinkle with salt or onion powder and dill.
5. Place on a plate and cook on high in a microwave oven for 30 to 45 seconds, or broil for 5 minutes.
6. Serve with grapes on the side.

Muffin
Calories: 111
Protein: 11 g
Fat: 0.9 g
Sodium: 363 mg
Cholesterol: 6 mg

Grapes
Calories: 57
Protein: 0.6 g
Fat: 0
Sodium: 2 mg
Cholesterol: 0

8. Poached Egg Push-Up with Raspberries

Serves 1

1 medium to large tomato
Sprinkle of salt
Sprinkle of oregano
1 slice whole wheat bread
1 egg
1 cup raspberries

1. Bring water to a boil in small saucepan.
2. Slice tomato and arrange in a circle on a plate. Sprinkle with salt and oregano.
3. Toast the whole wheat bread and place in the center of the plate.
4. Place the egg in boiling water and cook 30 to 45 seconds, to soft boil. Watch the egg; you don't want the yellow to turn hard.
5. Scoop egg out of shell onto the toast.
6. Serve with raspberries on the side.

Egg
Calories: 161
Protein: 9.7 g
Fat: 6.3 g
Sodium: 314 mg
Cholesterol: 265 mg

Raspberries
Calories: 109
Protein: 2.3 g
Fat: 2.1 g
Sodium: 1 mg
Cholesterol: 0

9. Joyce's Red, White, and Blue Delight

Serves 1

4 eggs
1 large tomato
1 large red bell pepper
3 large romaine lettuce leaves
Sprinkle of garlic-flavored wine vinegar
¼ teaspoon salt (or onion powder)
1 cup blueberries

1. Boil eggs for 7 minutes until hard-boiled.
2. While eggs are boiling, slice tomato. Cut red pepper into rings and strips, and arrange over lettuce leaves.
3. Sprinkle with vinegar and salt or onion powder.
4. When eggs are cooked, place in a pot of cold water to cool and remove the shells.
5. Separate whites from yolks and discard yolks.
6. Cut whites into rings and strips and arrange in center of tomato-pepper mixture.
7. Sprinkle with salt or onion powder and serve with blueberries on the side.

Eggs
Calories: 117
Protein: 15 g
Fat: 0.6 g
Sodium: 204 mg
Cholesterol: 0

Blueberries
Calories: 89
Protein: 1.1 g
Fat: 0.6 g
Sodium: 10 mg
Cholesterol: 0

10. Energy Egg Drop Soup with Kiwi

Serves 1

1 cup water
1 cup low-sodium chicken broth
Pinch of parsley flakes
1 egg
⅛ teaspoon salt (or onion powder)
1 slice whole wheat bread
1 large or 2 small kiwi fruit

1. Boil water and add chicken broth and parsley flakes.
2. Beat egg until thoroughly mixed.
3. Pour egg slowly into water while, with the other hand, stirring with a fork. Continue stirring the boiling mixture for about 15 seconds. Season with salt.
4. Pour soup into a cup or bowl and dip bread into the soup.
5. Serve with kiwi fruit on the side.

Soup
Calories: 146
Protein: 11 g
Fat: 6 g
Sodium: 467 mg
Cholesterol: 265 mg

Kiwi Fruit
Calories: 80
Protein: 1.2 g
Fat: 0.5 g
Sodium: 7 mg
Cholesterol: 0

ULTRA-QUICKIE BREAKFASTS

These recipes are for those who must eat walking out the door or else miss breakfast! I'm not even numbering these because they're so quick I'm not counting them. They are a bonus.

2 Slices Whole Wheat Toast

Calories: 112
Protein: 4.8 g
Fat: 1.4 g
Sodium: 242 mg
Cholesterol: 1 mg

1 Baked Potato

Bake it the night before.

Calories: 217
Protein: 6 g
Fat: 0
Sodium: 9 mg
Cholesterol: 0

1 Cup of Raisin Bran Cereal

Pour into a Baggy and eat like candy.

Calories: 177
Protein: 6.2 g
Fat: 1.2 g
Sodium: 414 mg
Cholesterol: 0

8 Ounces Low-Fat Yogurt and 3 Low-Fat Melba Rounds

Calories: 179
Protein: 15 g
Fat: 0.2 g
Sodium: 171 mg
Cholesterol: 5 mg

1 Ounce Pretzels

Choose regular or low-sodium pretzels with 1 gram or less fat.

Calories: 110
Protein: 4 g
Fat: 1 g
Sodium: 10 mg
Cholesterol: 0

1 Serving SnackWell's Cinnamon Graham Snacks

Calories: 110
Protein: 2 g
Fat: 0
Sodium: 90 mg
Cholesterol: 0

½ Sara Lee 97% Fat Free Sesame Seed Bagel

Maybe take a small tomato to wet your whistle.

Calories: 105
Protein: 4.0 g
Fat: 1.4 g
Sodium: 265 mg
Cholesterol: 0

What about a piece of fruit and nothing else in the morning? Not a great idea! It will give you a quick energy boost and a soon-to-come letdown. Have some complex carbohydrates with the fruit.

NOT-QUITE-AS-QUICK BREAKFASTS

Okay, let's resume the numbers. The following breakfasts take a little longer to make but they are worth it.

11. Catch-Me-If-You-Can Cornbread Crunch with Cantaloupe

Serves 8; makes 16 slices, 2 slices per serving

1 cup yellow cornmeal
1 cup whole wheat flour
1 tablespoon baking powder
10 packets artificial sweetener (optional)
1 cup skim milk
1 tablespoon lemon juice
1 tablespoon apple juice concentrate
2 egg whites
2 tablespoons applesauce
¼ cantaloupe

1. Preheat oven to 400°F.
2. In a large mixing bowl, thoroughly combine cornmeal, flour, baking powder, and artificial sweetener.
3. In another bowl, combine skim milk, lemon juice, apple juice concentrate, egg whites, and applesauce and mix thoroughly.
4. Add milk mixture to cornmeal mixture, blending thoroughly. Pour the batter into an 8-inch nonstick baking pan.
5. Bake for 25 minutes, or until the top turns golden brown. Cut into 16 slices. Serve 2 slices with ¼ cantaloupe.

Cornbread (2)
Calories: 122
Protein: 5.2 g
Fat: 0.8 g
Sodium: 159 mg
Cholesterol: 1 mg

Cantaloupe
Calories: 35
Protein: 0.9 g
Fat: 0
Sodium: 9 mg
Cholesterol: 0

12. Giant-Set Tomato-Cucumber Crepes with Orange Wedges

Serves 8; makes 4 crepes, ½ crepe per serving

½ cup skim milk
2 egg whites
½ cup whole wheat flour
⅛ teaspoon celery seed
4 small tomatoes, diced
2 small cucumbers, diced
2 tablespoons wine vinegar (or more; optional)
⅛ teaspoon onion powder
⅛ teaspoon oregano
Salt (optional)
8 small navel oranges, separated into wedges
2⅔ cups granola (Nature Valley)

1. Combine the milk, egg whites, flour, and celery seed in a food processor or blender until thoroughly mixed.
2. Spoon 2 tablespoons of batter onto a very hot nonstick skillet, quickly spreading batter (you may roll the pan from side to side) until it covers entire pan.
3. When edges of crepe have curled, turn and brown other side.

4. Make the rest of the crepes in the same manner.

5. Place diced tomatoes and cucumbers in a small bowl and add the vinegar, onion powder, and oregano. (If using, sprinkle salt to taste.)

6. Divide tomato-cucumber mixture into four parts, place in center of each crepe, and roll up. Fasten crepes closed with toothpicks and cut into halves.

7. Place crepe halves on individual salad plates and circle with orange wedges.

8. Sprinkle with ⅓ cup granola.

Crepes
Calories: 54
Protein: 3 g
Fat: 0.3 g
Sodium: 24 mg
Cholesterol: 0

Orange Wedges
Calories: 69
Protein: 1.5 g
Fat: 0.1 g
Sodium: 2 mg
Cholesterol: 0

Granola (Nature Valley)
Calories: 126
Protein: 2.9 g
Fat: 4.9 g
Sodium: 58 mg
Cholesterol: 0

13. Spicy Superset Omelet and Toast

Serves 2

½ cup chopped onion
¼ cup chopped red bell pepper
¼ cup chopped green bell pepper
1 garlic clove, minced (or ½ teaspoon garlic powder)
6 small plum tomatoes, chopped
⅛ cup diced green chilies
1 6-ounce can low-sodium V-8 juice
½ teaspoon salt (optional)
⅛ teaspoon black pepper
½ teaspoon chili powder
½ teaspoon oregano
4 egg whites
4 slices whole wheat toast

1. In a large bowl, combine onion, peppers, garlic, tomatoes, chilies, juice, and all seasonings. Mix thoroughly.

2. Cook mixture in nonstick pan for 6 minutes over high heat, stirring often.

3. While the onion-pepper mixture is cooking, beat egg whites for about 20 seconds.

4. Fold onion-pepper mixture into egg whites and combine thoroughly.

5. Pour batter into a nonstick frying pan and cook until slightly brown on each side.

6. Serve with toast.

Omelet
Calories: 176
Protein: 12 g
Fat: 0.7 g
Sodium: 195 mg
Cholesterol: 0

Whole Wheat Toast (2)
Calories: 112
Protein: 4.8 g
Fat: 1.4 g
Sodium: 242 mg
Cholesterol: 1 mg

14. Pita Pockets Power Omelet

Serves 1

½ red bell pepper, chopped
1 small plum tomato, chopped
½ small onion, chopped
3 mushrooms, chopped
3 tablespoons water
2 egg whites
⅛ teaspoon onion powder (or salt)
⅛ teaspoon garlic powder
1 whole wheat pita bread

1. Combine the red pepper, tomato, onion, mushrooms, and water.
2. Sauté in a nonstick frying pan for 6 minutes.
3. While pepper-mushroom mixture is cooking, beat egg whites for about 15 seconds, adding onion powder or salt and garlic powder as you beat.
4. Combine pepper mixture with egg whites and mix thoroughly. Pour mixture into a hot nonstick frying pan and cook about 1 minute on each side, or until slightly browned.
5. Stuff omelet into pita bread. You will have some omelet left over to put on the side of your plate and eat as an extra delight.

Calories: 196
Protein: 14 g
Fat: 1.3 g
Sodium: 321 mg
Cholesterol: 0

15. Joyce's Russian-French Toast

Serves 1

2 egg whites and 1 yolk
¼ cup skim milk
2 slices pumpernickel bread (or whole wheat bread)
½ cup nonfat plain yogurt (or fruit yogurt)
Generous sprinkling of onion powder

1. Beat yolk and whites with a fork for 10 seconds, then stir in milk until blended.
2. Dip bread into the mixture until thoroughly soaked on both sides.
3. Place bread in a nonstick frying pan over medium heat. Cover and cook until browned on both sides, turning over once or twice.
4. Coat the hot bread with the yogurt and sprinkle with onion powder.

Calories: 245
Protein: 20 g
Fat: 5.4 g
Sodium: 404 mg
Cholesterol: 225 mg

16. Nutty Nutmeg French Toast

Serves 2; makes 4 slices, 2 slices per serving

⅔ cup skim milk
1 tablespoon plain vinegar
4 egg whites
⅛ teaspoon nutmeg
⅛ teaspoon cinnamon
4 slices whole wheat bread
½ cup warmed applesauce

1. In a large bowl, mix milk, vinegar, egg whites, nutmeg, and cinnamon until ingredients are thoroughly combined.
2. Dip each slice of bread into the mixture, one at a time, piercing a few times with a fork so it can absorb the liquid. Let each slice soak for about 10 seconds.
3. Place the soaked bread in a hot nonstick frying pan and cook until golden brown on each side.
4. Spoon 1 tablespoon of warm applesauce onto each slice and sprinkle with cinnamon. (If desired, sprinkle the toast with artificial sweetener instead.)

Calories: 163
Protein: 12 g
Fat: 1.6 g
Sodium: 353 mg
Cholesterol: 3 mg

17. Eye-Opener Orange-Apple Muffins with Fruit

Serves 3; makes 6 muffins, 2 muffins per serving

¾ cup whole wheat flour
2 teaspoons baking powder
1½ cups oat bran cereal

1 cup orange juice
2 tablespoons apple juice concentrate (plus 9 packets artificial
   sweetener, optional)
⅛ teaspoon grated orange peel
1½ tablespoons applesauce
2 egg whites
3 cups fresh apple and orange wedges

1. Preheat oven to 400°F.

2. Mix together flour and baking powder and place on the side.

3. Combine cereal, orange juice, apple juice concentrate and optional sweetener, orange peel, applesauce, and egg whites.

4. Beat until thoroughly mixed, then add flour mixture and stir until fully blended.

5. Spoon evenly into a nonstick 6-muffin tin.

6. Bake for 25 minutes, or until tester comes out clean.

7. Serve surrounded by an array of apple and orange sections.

Muffins (2)
Calories: 170
Protein: 6.7 g
Fat: 0.5 g
Sodium: 266 mg
Cholesterol: 0

Orange and Apple Wedges
Calories: 97
Protein: 1.2 g
Fat: 0.4 g
Sodium: 2 mg
Cholesterol: 0

18. Call-the-Police Carrot Muffins with Applesauce

Serves 2; makes 4 muffins, 2 muffins per serving

2 egg whites
½ cup plain nonfat yogurt
1 tablespoon apple juice concentrate (plus 6 packets artificial
  sweetener, optional)
½ tablespoon applesauce, plus 1 cup applesauce for serving
⅓ cup shredded carrots
¾ cup whole wheat flour
1 teaspoon baking powder
⅛ teaspoon cinnamon
⅛ teaspoon salt (or celery seed)

1. Preheat oven to 375°F.
2. In a small bowl, beat egg whites until nearly stiff.
3. Fold in yogurt, apple juice concentrate, ½ tablespoon applesauce, and shredded carrots.
4. In a separate bowl, combine flour, baking powder, cinnamon, and salt or celery seed.
5. Stir egg whites into flour mixture and blend until evenly mixed.
6. Spoon batter into a 6-cup nonstick muffin pan. Bake for 15 minutes, or until tester comes out clean.
7. Serve with applesauce on the side.

Muffins (2)
Calories: 151
Protein: 8.7 g
Fat: 0.6 g
Sodium: 229 mg
Cholesterol: 0.8 mg

Applesauce
Calories: 50
Protein: 0.2 g

Fat: 0.2 g
Sodium: 3 mg
Cholesterol: 0

Note: You may want to triple the recipe and make an even dozen.

If not, fill the unused muffin wells with ⅓ cup water.

19. Barbell Banana-Almond-Raisin Muffins with Sliced Banana

Serves 3; makes 6 muffins, 2 muffins per serving

1 egg white
1 cup whole wheat flour
½ cup bran flakes
½ cup old-fashioned oats
¾ teaspoon baking soda
⅛ teaspoon nutmeg
⅓ cup apple juice concentrate
⅛ teaspoon almond extract
¼ cup plain nonfat yogurt
½ cup mashed banana
½ cup raisins
3 bananas, sliced
Sprinkle of nutmeg
Sprinkle of cinnamon

1. Preheat oven to 400°F.
2. Beat egg white in a small bowl until stiff and set aside.
3. In a separate bowl, mix flour, bran flakes, oats, baking soda, and nutmeg.
4. Fold the apple juice concentrate, almond extract, yogurt, banana, and raisins into flour mixture.
5. Fold in the egg white and stir until thoroughly combined.
6. Spoon the batter into a 6-cup nonstick muffin pan. Bake for 20 minutes, or until tester comes out clean.
7. Serve with sliced bananas sprinkled with nutmeg and cinnamon.

Note: You may experiment with this recipe by replacing the extract with any extract of your choice.

Muffins (2)
Calories: 348
Protein: 12 g
Fat: 1.9 g
Sodium: 243 mg
Cholesterol: 0

Sliced Bananas and Cinnamon
Calories: 139
Protein: 1.5 g
Fat: 0.8 g
Sodium: 2 mg
Cholesterol: 0

20. Pineapple Perk-Up Muffins with Pineapple Chunks

Serves 3; makes 6 muffins, 2 muffins per serving

2 egg whites
⅛ teaspoon vanilla extract
⅛ teaspoon lemon extract
½ cup bran cereal
¼ cup skim milk
⅛ cup applesauce
½ cup whole wheat flour
½ tablespoon baking powder
¼ teaspoon salt (or celery seed)
¾ tablespoon brown sugar
4 ounces undrained crushed canned pineapple (packed in unsweetened juice)
12 ounces drained unsweetened pineapple chunks, or 3 large slices fresh pineapple, cut into eighths

1. Preheat oven to 400°F.

2. In a small bowl, beat egg whites slightly and fold in vanilla and lemon extracts.

3. Fold in cereal, milk, and applesauce and set aside.

4. In a separate bowl, combine the flour, baking powder, salt, and brown sugar and stir well.

5. Stir egg white mixture into dry mixture and mix thoroughly.

6. Fold in the crushed pineapple and its juice.

7. Spoon into a 6-cup nonstick muffin pan. Bake for 22 minutes, or until tester comes out clean.

8. Serve with ½ cup pineapple chunks or pineapple slice.

Muffins (2)
Calories: 149
Protein: 6.7 g
Fat: 0.9 g
Sodium: 281 mg
Cholesterol: 0

Pineapple
Calories: 68
Protein: 0.4 g
Fat: 0.1 g
Sodium: 1 mg
Cholesterol: 0

21. Aerobic Bran-Apple Muffins with Stuffed Apple

Serves 3; makes 6 muffins, 2 muffins per serving

½ cup whole wheat flour
½ teaspoon baking soda
⅛ teaspoon salt (or celery seed)
¾ cup wheat bran
2 tablespoons plus ¾ cup applesauce
¼ cup molasses
¾ cup buttermilk
½ cup diced apple
3 apples, cored
Sprinkle of cinnamon

1. Preheat oven to 375°F.
2. Combine flour, baking soda, salt, and wheat bran and mix thoroughly.
3. Fold in 2 tablespoons applesauce, molasses, and buttermilk and mix well.
4. Fold in diced apple and mix thoroughly.
5. Spoon batter into a 6-cup nonstick muffin pan. Bake for 15 minutes, or until tester comes out clean.
6. Spoon ¼ cup applesauce into each apple and sprinkle with cinnamon. Serve stuffed apples with muffins.

Muffins (2)
Calories: 152
Protein: 4 g
Fat: 0.7 g
Sodium: 167 mg
Cholesterol: 1 mg

Stuffed Apple
Calories: 114
Protein: 0
Fat: 0.7 g

Sodium: 3 mg
Cholesterol: 0

22. Bella Russia Potato Pancakes and Sour Cream with an Apple

Serves 3; makes 6 pancakes, 2 pancakes per serving

2 egg whites
½ cup skim milk
2 peeled baked potatoes
⅓ cup plain bread crumbs
¼ teaspoon salt
½ teaspoon onion powder
1 cup nonfat sour cream
3 medium apples

1. Beat the egg whites for about 30 seconds and set aside.
2. Using milk as needed, mash potatoes thoroughly and add beaten egg whites.
3. Fold in bread crumbs, salt, and onion powder.
4. Using about ¼ cup per pancake, spoon batter into a hot nonstick skillet and cook until bubbles form in the center of the pancake and the frying side is golden brown. Turn over and cook until the other side is golden brown.
5. Serve each pancake with a heaping tablespoon of sour cream on top and an apple on the side.

Note: You can make these pancakes bigger by using ⅓ to ½ cup batter. Of course, you will have fewer pancakes this way.

Pancakes (2)
Calories: 270
Protein: 14 g
Fat: 0.6 g
Sodium: 308 mg
Cholesterol: 1 mg

Apple
Calories: 89
Protein: 20 g
Fat: 0.6 g
Sodium: 2 mg
Cholesterol: 0

23. Busy Bee Banana-Strawberry Pancakes with Sliced Strawberries

Serves 3; makes 6 pancakes, 2 pancakes per serving

1 large overripe banana
4 egg whites
⅛ teaspoon vanilla extract
1 cup whole wheat flour
¼ cup water
½ cup instant oatmeal
4 large strawberries

1. Mash banana in a bowl.
2. Mix in egg whites, vanilla, flour, water, and oatmeal and set aside until mixture has solidified, about 2 minutes.
3. Using about ⅓ cup per pancake, spoon the batter into a hot nonstick skillet and cook until bubbles form in the center of the pancake and the frying side is golden brown. Turn over and cook until the other side is golden brown.
4. Slice the strawberries and place on top of the pancakes.

Pancakes (2)
Calories: 299
Protein: 12 g
Fat: 1.7 g
Sodium: 65 mg
Cholesterol: 0

Strawberries
Calories: 45
Protein: 0.9 g
Fat: 0.6 g
Sodium: 2 mg
Cholesterol: 0

24. Buckeye Opener Pancakes with Apricots

Serves 3; makes 9 pancakes, 3 pancakes per serving

2 egg whites
1 tablespoon apple juice concentrate
⅔ cup nonfat buttermilk
1 tablespoon applesauce
½ cup buckwheat flour
¼ cup whole wheat flour
1 teaspoon baking powder
½ teaspoon baking soda
¼ teaspoon salt (or onion powder)
12 dried apricots

1. Combine the egg whites, apple juice concentrate, and buttermilk. Beat until well blended.

2. Fold in the applesauce, flours, baking powder, baking soda, and salt. Mix thoroughly.

3. Make small pancakes by dropping a generous tablespoon of batter into a hot nonstick frying pan and brown until bubbles appear in the middle of the pancake and edges turn up. Flip and brown on other side.

4. Serve with 4 apricots per serving.

Pancakes (3)
Calories: 118
Protein: 5.3 g
Fat: 0.6 g
Sodium: 306 mg
Cholesterol: 1 mg

Apricots
Calories: 26
Protein: 0.4 g
Fat: 0
Sodium: 1 mg
Cholesterol: 0

25. Blueberry Wheat Wake-Up Pancakes with Blueberries

Serves 2; makes 4 pancakes, 2 pancakes per serving

½ cup whole wheat flour
½ teaspoon baking powder
¼ teaspoon baking soda
¾ cup skim milk
⅛ teaspoon vanilla extract
2½ cups blueberries

1. Combine flour, baking powder, and baking soda and set aside.
2. In a large bowl, mix skim milk and vanilla.
3. Stir in flour combination and mix until fully blended.
4. Fold in ½ cup of blueberries and mix until thoroughly blended.
5. Using about ¼ cup per pancake, spoon batter into a hot nonstick skillet and cook until bubbles form in the center of the pancake and the frying side is golden brown. Turn over and cook until the other side is golden brown.
6. Serve with remaining 2 cups blueberries on the side.

Pancakes (2)
Calories: 155
Protein: 7.6 g
Fat: 0.9 g
Sodium: 241 mg
Cholesterol: 2 mg

Blueberries
Calories: 89
Protein: 1.1 g
Fat: 0.6 g
Sodium: 10 mg
Cholesterol: 0

26. Raisin Oatmeal Rise-and-Shine Pancakes with Raspberries

Serves 3; makes 6 pancakes, 2 pancakes per serving

¾ cup old-fashioned oats
¾ cup nonfat buttermilk
½ teaspoon baking soda
¼ cup whole wheat flour
2 tablespoons apple juice concentrate
½ teaspoon almond extract
1 egg white
½ cup raisins
3 cups raspberries

1. Pour oats into a blender or food processor and chop until fully ground. (You will need the chopping blade for this.)
2. Add buttermilk, baking soda, flour, apple juice concentrate, almond extract, and egg white and fully blend.
3. Remove batter from blender or food processor and fold in raisins.
4. Using about ¼ cup per pancake, spoon batter into a hot nonstick skillet and cook until bubbles form in the center of the pancake and the frying side is golden brown. Turn over and cook until the other side is golden brown.
5. Serve with raspberries on the side.

Note: If you don't want to use a food processor or blender, substitute ⅔ cup whole oat flour for the oats and simply mix ingredients in a bowl in the same order.

Pancakes (2)
Calories: 224
Protein: 7.6 g
Fat: 1.9 g
Sodium: 182 mg
Cholesterol: 1 mg

Raspberries
Calories: 109
Protein: 2.3 g
Fat: 2.1 g
Sodium: 1 mg
Cholesterol: 0

27. Jumping Gingerbread-Nutmeg Apple Pancakes with Apples

Serves 3; makes 6 pancakes, 2 pancakes per serving

½ cup whole wheat flour
¼ teaspoon baking soda
¼ teaspoon ginger
⅛ teaspoon cinnamon
⅛ teaspoon nutmeg
⅛ teaspoon onion powder
⅛ teaspoon ground cloves
2 egg whites
4 ounces apple juice concentrate
⅛ teaspoon vanilla extract
1 tablespoon applesauce
3 apples, cut into wedges

1. In a large mixing bowl, combine flour, baking soda, ginger, cinnamon, nutmeg, onion powder, and cloves.
2. In another bowl, beat egg whites for 30 seconds.
3. Fold apple juice concentrate, vanilla, and applesauce into the egg whites.

4. Combine the flour mixture with the egg white mixture, mixing until fully combined but lumpy.

5. Using about ¼ cup per pancake, spoon batter into a hot nonstick frying pan and cook until bubbles form in the center of the pancake and the frying side is golden brown. Turn over and cook until the other side is golden brown.

6. Serve surrounded by apple wedges.

Pancakes (2)
Calories: 131
Protein: 5.6 g
Fat: 0.5 g
Sodium: 137 mg
Cholesterol: 0

Apple Wedges
Calories: 89
Protein: 0
Fat: 0.6 g
Sodium: 2 mg
Cholesterol: 0

28. Biceps Buttermilk Pancakes with Tangerines and Milk

Serves 3; makes 6 pancakes, 2 pancakes per serving

2 egg whites
⅛ teaspoon baking soda
¼ teaspoon onion powder
½ cup skim milk (optional; see Note)
2 teaspoons lemon juice
1 teaspoon applesauce
½ cup whole wheat flour
9 tangerines, separated into wedges
1 glass 1% milk

1. Mix egg whites in a large bowl until nearly stiff.

2. Add in baking soda and onion powder and beat until foamy.

3. Mix in milk, lemon juice, and applesauce and combine thoroughly.

4. Fold in flour and mix well.

5. Using about ¼ cup per pancake, spoon the batter into a hot nonstick skillet and cook until bubbles form in the center of the pancake and the frying side is golden brown. Turn over and cook until the other side is golden brown.

6. Serve with tangerine wedges and a glass of milk.

Note: You can use buttermilk for a double whammy, but the lemon juice sours the milk anyway.

Pancakes (2)
Calories: 93
Protein: 6.3 g
Fat: 0
Sodium: 88 mg
Cholesterol: 0.8 mg

Tangerine Wedges
Calories: 66
Protein: 0.9 g
Fat: 0
Sodium: 2 mg
Cholesterol: 0

Glass of 1% Milk
Calories: 102
Protein: 8 g
Fat: 2.6 g
Sodium: 123 mg
Cholesterol: 10 mg

29. Popeye's Wake-Up Pizza with Papaya

Serves 1

1 large tomato, sliced
2 slices whole wheat bread
2 1-ounce slices low-fat mozzarella cheese
⅛ teaspoon garlic powder
⅛ teaspoon oregano
Sprinkle of salt (optional)
1 cup papaya cubes

1. Place a few slices tomatoes on each piece of bread. Save 1 slice each for top of cheese.
2. Cover tomatoes with cheese.
3. Place 1 tomato slice on top of each "pizza."
4. Sprinkle with garlic powder, oregano, and salt.
5. Place on a plate and cook uncovered on high in a microwave oven for 45 seconds to a minute, or in a broiler for about 5 minutes.
6. Serve with papaya.

Pizzas (2)
Calories: 223
Protein: 23 g
Fat: 11 g
Sodium: 176 mg
Cholesterol: 11 mg

Papaya
Calories: 104
Protein: 1.6 g
Fat: 0
Sodium: 8 mg
Cholesterol: 0

30. Power Potato-Plum Energy Breakfast

Serves 1

½ lemon
2 medium new potatoes, cut into 8 parts
⅛ teaspoon garlic powder
⅛ teaspoon onion powder
⅛ teaspoon paprika
⅛ teaspoon oregano
Sprinkle of black pepper
Sprinkle of crushed red pepper
2 plums

1. Squeeze lemon juice onto the potatoes.
2. Sprinkle with garlic powder, onion powder, paprika, oregano, pepper, and red pepper.
3. Place on a plate and cook on high in a microwave oven for 5 to 6 minutes (check to see if soft), or in standard oven for 25 minutes.
4. Serve with 2 plums on the side.

Potatoes
Calories: 140
Protein: 3.1 g
Fat: 0
Sodium: 10 mg
Cholesterol: 0

Plums
Calories: 66
Protein: 0.5 g
Fat: 0
Sodium: 2 mg
Cholesterol: 0

31. Slavic Stuffed Baked Potato with Honeydew

Serves 1

1 medium to large baking potato
¼ cup nonfat cottage cheese
⅛ cup nonfat plain yogurt or nonfat sour cream
Sprinkle of garlic powder
Sprinkle of onion powder
Sprinkle of salt
Sprinkle of paprika
¼ honeydew melon

1. Place potato on a plate and cook on high in a microwave oven for 6 to 7 minutes (check to see if soft), or bake for 45 minutes in standard oven.

2. While potato is cooking, combine cottage cheese, yogurt or sour cream, garlic powder, onion powder, and salt and mix well.

3. Remove the insides of the baked potato.

4. Fill the potato with cottage cheese mixture and sprinkle with paprika.

5. Return potato to microwave oven for 25 seconds or standard oven for 10 minutes.

6. Serve with wedge of honeydew.

Potato
Calories: 250
Protein: 8 g
Fat: 0.3 g
Sodium: 49 mg
Cholesterol: 0

Honeydew
Calories: 53
Protein: 0.8 g
Fat: 0
Sodium: 15 mg
Cholesterol: 0

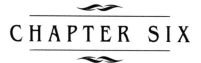

CHAPTER SIX

LUNCH MENUS FOR A MONTH

Whether we work at home or in an office, the lunch break is for most of us a carrot on a stick—something that we look forward to, something that keeps us going. We all look forward to lunch! But believe it or not, some people skip lunch. Foolishly, they think, "I'd rather not stop my work and waste time with lunch." But they are wrong. Skipping lunch will cause them to work less efficiently, and with less energy, they may well waste more time than if they had stopped for lunch. In addition, if they are trying to lose weight, skipping meals will only slow the process down.

The following pages contain a month's worth of lunches. The first ten recipes will take less time to prepare than the twenty-one lunches that follow; however, even the longer recipes do not take very long. Also, at the end of the chapter I give you seven bonus soups that take a moderate amount of time to prepare, but can be prepared ahead of time and refrigerated.

UNDERSTANDING THE NUTRITIONAL INFORMATION

Following each recipe are one or more nutritional analyses listing the calorie content plus protein, fat, sodium, and carbohydrate found in the food. The calculations are *per serving* unless otherwise indicated. For example, in a recipe serving four persons, the analysis will be for one serving. For a recipe yielding six patties, two patties constituting a serving, the analysis will be for two patties.

You will note that when fruit or a vegetable is added as a side dish, the calculations are shown separately—one analysis for the main dish and one for the side dish—so that you have detailed information on the food values of the specific foods you are eating. Also, if you are using the recipes to make up your own meal plans, you might want to eliminate or substitute the side dish.

Protein and fat measures are shown in grams (g); sodium and carbohydrate contents are given in milligrams (mg). Refer to Chapter 3 for guidelines on using these figures. Bear in mind, however, that the meal plans in Chapter 9 count everything for you—these analyses are for your information in case you want to make your own daily meal plans.

When an alternative ingredient appears in parentheses, this means the substitute has not been included in the analysis. For example, "1 teaspoon garlic powder (or salt)" means that the analysis includes garlic powder but not salt (which would yield a higher sodium content).

When recipes include wheat germ or canola oil, the analysis for these items is usually kept separate. I've added these items in the recipe to meet the fat requirements in the meal plans, but if you are developing your own meal plans, you might want to omit these items and obtain your fat minimum in another way. In the rare cases when it is included in the recipe, it is because I feel it is absolutely necessary to the taste of the recipe.

A NOTE ABOUT THE RECIPES

Where nonstick cookware is involved, it is assumed that you have lightly coated the cookware with a vegetable oil cooking spray, like Pam.

When 1 percent dairy products are used, feel free to substitute nonfat products. I use the 1 percent items when I feel you need that bit of fat to fulfill a healthy daily fat requirement. (The minimum fat you should get is 10 percent of total caloric intake.)

Feel free to substitute the fruit or vegetable on the side with any other fruit or vegetable, or eliminate the item at the meal and eat it any other time of the day. Just be sure to replace side-dish vegetable suggestions with vegetables from the equivalent lists in Chapter 3. In other words, you must replace unlimited complex carbohydrate vegetables with unlimited and limited with limited. Also, if you don't want to eat as much of the vegetable as is suggested, you can cut the quantity, but be sure that you still get your bare minimum of 3 cups of vegetables for the day. You can, of course, also eat more of the unlimited complex carbohydrate vegetables if you desire. Also feel free to cut the serving size in half if you feel it is too much for you. For example, sometimes I give you two sandwiches for lunch. I do this because I have no trouble eating such portions. But you're not me, so do what suits you best.

Fruits and vegetables in the ingredients lists are medium size unless otherwise indicated. Herbs and spices are dried unless fresh is indicated.

10 QUICKIE LUNCHES

1. Kiev Cottage Cheese and Pumpernickel Sandwich and Salad

Serves 1

½ cup low-fat cottage cheese
4 tablespoons nonfat sour cream
2 slices pumpernickel bread
½ cucumber, thinly sliced
Sprinkle of dill
¼ head lettuce
1 large tomato, cut into eighths
Flavored vinegar
Sprinkle of onion powder (or salt)

1. Mix cottage cheese with sour cream.
2. Spread mixture onto pumpernickel bread. Add cucumber slices and sprinkle with dill.
3. Close sandwich with other slice of bread.
4. Break up lettuce in a small bowl and add tomatoes. Sprinkle with vinegar and onion powder and serve.

Sandwich
Calories: 307
Protein: 24 g
Fat: 2.1 g
Sodium: 908 mg
Cholesterol: 6 mg

Salad
Calories: 45
Protein: 2.2 g
Fat: 0.5 g
Sodium: 9 mg
Cholesterol: 0

2. Tangy Tuna-Cucumber-Onion Sandwich on Whole Wheat with Red Peppers and Tomatoes

Serves 1—a big lunch

4 ounces tuna packed in water, rinsed and drained
1 tablespoon nonfat mayonnaise
½ cucumber, diced
½ onion, diced
2 large lettuce leaves
4 slices whole wheat bread
1 large tomato, sliced
1 large red pepper, sliced
Garlic-flavored wine vinegar
Pinch of salt (optional)

1. In a small bowl, break up tuna with a fork and mix in mayonnaise. Add cucumber and onion and mix thoroughly.
2. Place lettuce leaves on 2 slices of bread.
3. Divide tuna mixture in half and place on lettuce leaves. Close sandwich with other slice of bread.
4. Arrange tomato and red pepper on a large plate and sprinkle with vinegar and salt.

Sandwiches (2)
Calories: 395
Protein: 37 g
Fat: 5.1 g
Sodium: 555 mg
Cholesterol: 43 mg

Red Peppers and Tomatoes
Calories: 40
Protein: 2 g
Fat: 0.4 g
Sodium: 10 mg
Cholesterol: 0

3. Luscious Lettuce and Tomato Sandwich with Vegetables

Serves 1

4 slices whole wheat bread, toasted
3 tablespoons nonfat mayonnaise
¼ head lettuce
1 large tomato, sliced
Sprinkle of salt
2 cups broccoli and cauliflower mix, from frozen package,
　　cooked

1. Coat both slices of toast very generously with mayonnaise.
2. Place a large lettuce leaf on top of mayonnaise and cover
with tomato slices.
3. Sprinkle with salt and close the sandwich with the other
slice of bread.
4. Serve with a bowl of broccoli and cauliflower.

Sandwiches (2)
Calories: 313
Protein: 12 g
Fat: 3.3 g
Sodium: 617 mg
Cholesterol: 3 mg

Broccoli and Cauliflower
Calories: 97
Protein: 10 g
Fat: 1 g
Sodium: 52 mg
Cholesterol: 0

4. Jump-Start Soup and Such

Serves 1

1 16-ounce can Progresso Healthy Classics Chicken Noodle
   Soup (or similar soup)
2 slices whole wheat bread
1 cup large strawberry slices
3 large lettuce leaves
1 package artificial sweetener (optional)

1. Place soup in a pot. Break up bread into small pieces and throw into the soup. Heat the soup until piping hot.

2. Arrange sliced strawberries over lettuce leaves. Sprinkle with sweetener.

3. Serve on the side with the soup

Note: The soup will turn into a delicious, thick porridge. Yes, you get to eat the whole can, not the tiny amount they call a "serving."

Soup
Calories: 261
Protein: 13 g
Fat: 6.2 g
Sodium: 1040 mg
Cholesterol: 40 mg

Strawberries
Calories: 61
Protein: 1.9 g
Fat: 0.8 g
Sodium: 8 mg
Cholesterol: 0

5. Tantalizing Tuna Toss and Toast

Serves 1

4 ounces tuna packed in water, rinsed and drained
½ head lettuce
2 tomatoes, cut into eighths
1 cucumber, diced
1 onion, halved and thinly sliced
1 red bell pepper, diced or slivered
Wine vinegar
Sprinkle of oregano
Sprinkle of pepper
Sprinkle of salt (optional)
1 slice whole wheat bread, toasted

1. In a small bowl, break up tuna and set aside.
2. In a large bowl, break up lettuce and add tomatoes, cucumber, onion, and red pepper. Add tuna and mix thoroughly. Add plenty of vinegar to taste and toss thoroughly. Sprinkle with oregano, pepper, and salt.
3. Serve with toast on the side.

Tuna
Calories: 262
Protein: 33 g
Fat: 3.3 g
Sodium: 93 mg
Cholesterol: 40 mg

Toast
Calories: 56
Protein: 2.4 g
Fat: 0.7 g
Sodium: 121 mg
Cholesterol: 1 mg

6. Yogurt and Fruit Fiesta with English Bran Muffin and Milk

Serves 1

½ cantaloupe
4 ounces fruit-flavored low-fat yogurt
½ cup blueberries
½ English bran muffin, toasted and spread with 1 tablespoon fruit jam
1 glass 1% milk

1. Seed the halved cantaloupe and fill it with the yogurt.
2. Spread the berries along the side of the plate.
3. Quarter the muffin and arrange around the berries.
4. Serve with milk.

Cantaloupe
Calories: 226
Protein: 6.7 g
Fat: 2.2 g
Sodium: 83 mg
Cholesterol: 5 mg

Glass of Milk
Calories: 102
Protein: 8 g
Fat: 2.6 g
Sodium: 123 mg
Cholesterol: 10 mg

English Muffin and Strawberry Preserves
Calories: 110
Protein: 2.5 g
Fat: 0.7 g
Sodium: 124 mg
Cholesterol: 1 mg

7. Mmm Mmm Good Microwave Baked Potatoes and Cottage Cheese with Green Beans

Serves 1

2 baking potatoes
½ cup low-fat cottage cheese
Sprinkle of paprika
Sprinkle of onion powder
Sprinkle of salt (optional)
1 cup frozen green beans, cooked

1. Stab the potatoes in 8 places with a fork. Bake in microwave oven on high for 5 to 7 minutes (check to see if soft), or in standard oven for 45 minutes.

2. Cut off top end of potatoes and scoop out the insides, leaving enough space in each potato to fill with cottage cheese. Divide the cottage cheese into halves and stuff into potato shells.

3. Top with paprika, onion powder, and salt (if using).

4. Serve with green beans on the side.

Potatoes and Cheese
Calories: 516
Protein: 26 g
Fat: 1.8 g
Sodium: 478 mg
Cholesterol: 6 mg

Green Beans
Calories: 51
Protein: 3.2 g
Fat: 0.4 g
Sodium: 8 mg
Cholesterol: 0

8. Speed-Set Salmon Sandwich with Vegetables

Serves 1

4 ounces canned salmon, drained
2 scallions, cut up
1 tomato, diced
¼ onion, diced
Sprinkle of lemon juice
Sprinkle of dill
1 whole wheat pita bread
1 cup frozen carrots, cooked
Sprinkle of Butter Buds

1. In a small bowl, break up salmon. Add scallions, tomato, onion, and lemon juice and mix thoroughly. Sprinkle in dill and mix thoroughly.
2. Stuff into pita bread.
3. Serve with hot carrots sprinkled with Butter Buds and additional dill.

Sandwich
Calories: 328
Protein: 29 g
Fat: 7.8 g
Sodium: 294 mg
Cholesterol: 40 mg

Carrots
Calories: 47
Protein: 1.4 g
Fat: 0
Sodium: 50 mg
Cholesterol: 0

9. Turkey Trot on Toast with Green Beans

Serves 1

2 slices whole wheat bread, toasted
1 tablespoon mustard
1 large lettuce leaf
4 ounces sliced turkey breast
1 large tomato, sliced
½ large Spanish onion, thinly sliced
1 cucumber, thinly sliced
4 large mushrooms, thinly sliced
1 cup green beans, cooked

1. Spread both slices of toast with mustard and place a lettuce leaf on one of the slices. Add the turkey and 2 slices of tomato and onion, and close the sandwich.

2. Arrange the remaining lettuce leaves on a large plate and place the sandwich in the center of the leaves.

3. Arrange the remaining tomato slices, cucumber, remaining onion, and mushrooms in a pretty pattern around the plate and serve with green beans.

Sandwich
Calories: 393
Protein: 40 g
Fat: 5.7 g
Sodium: 542 mg
Cholesterol: 72 mg

Green Beans
Calories: 57
Protein: 3.2 g
Fat: 0.4 g
Sodium: 8 mg
Cholesterol: 0

10. End-All Egg Salad Sandwich with Stir-Fried Vegetables

Serves 1

3 eggs
¼ onion, chopped
2 tablespoons nonfat mayonnaise
⅛ teaspoon onion salt
Sprinkle of salt (optional)
Sprinkle of pepper
Sprinkle of parsley
1 large lettuce leaf
2 slices whole wheat bread, toasted
2 cups frozen stir-fried vegetables, cooked (see Note)

1. Boil the eggs until hard-boiled, about 7 minutes.
2. Remove the yolks from 2 eggs and discard. Chop the remaining yolk and egg whites into small pieces.
3. Add the chopped onion, mayonnaise, onion salt, salt, pepper, and parsley and mix thoroughly.
4. Place lettuce leaf on the whole wheat toast and spread the egg mixture on the lettuce. Close with the other slice of toast.
5. Serve with 2 cups of piping hot stir-fried vegetables.

Sandwich
Calories: 262
Protein: 18 g
Fat: 6.9 g
Sodium: 531 mg
Cholesterol: 266 mg

Stir-Fried Vegetables
Calories: 64
Protein: 6 g
Fat: 0.8 g
Sodium: 260 mg
Cholesterol: 0

Note: There should be no fat in the vegetables. The fat comes in when people fry the vegetables. Check when you buy the vegetables at the store.

OTHER LUNCHES

11. Dragon Lady's Spicy Rice and Vegetables

Serves 2

½ large onion, chopped
1 garlic clove, minced (or ⅛ teaspoon garlic powder)
1 large tomato, diced
1⅓ cups low-sodium chicken broth
½ teaspoon curry powder
⅛ teaspoon chili powder
⅛ teaspoon onion powder
½ cup uncooked instant brown rice
1 tablespoon chopped parsley
1 cup carrots, cooked
1 cup broccoli florets, cooked

1. "Sauté" the onion, garlic, and tomato in ⅓ cup chicken broth over very high heat until soft, about 2 minutes.
2. Add curry powder, chili powder, and onion powder and stir thoroughly.
3. Add remaining 1 cup of broth and rice and bring to a boil. Reduce heat to low and simmer, covered, for 5 minutes.
4. Let stand 5 minutes, then stir in parsley. Serve with carrots and broccoli on the side.

Rice
Calories: 167
Protein: 8.2 g
Fat: 1.1 g
Sodium: 141 mg
Cholesterol: 0

Broccoli
Calories: 52
Protein: 6.2 g
Fat: 0.6 g
Sodium: 20 mg
Cholesterol: 0

Carrots
Calories: 46
Protein: 1.4 g
Fat: 0
Sodium: 50 mg
Cholesterol: 0

12. Wonder Woman's White Wine Pasta with Salad

Serves 2

½ onion, thinly sliced
½ cup low-sodium chicken broth
1 scallion, minced
½ red bell pepper, finely chopped
1 cup diced yellow squash, cooked
⅔ cup dry white wine
1 tablespoon lemon juice
¼ cup chopped fresh parsley
¼ teaspoon oregano
¼ teaspoon basil
¼ teaspoon celery seed
¼ teaspoon garlic powder
⅛ teaspoon salt (or onion powder)
1½ cups cooked linguine
¼ head romaine lettuce
1 large tomato
2 tablespoons balsamic vinegar

1. "Sauté" onion in the broth over very high heat for about 3 minutes.

2. Add scallion and red pepper and cook for 3 more minutes, covered, over medium-high heat.

3. Fold in squash, mixing thoroughly. Add wine, lemon juice, and seasonings and mix until fully blended.

4. Mix in linguine and heat for about 30 seconds, stirring a couple of times.

5. Serve with a tossed salad of lettuce and tomato, dressed with balsamic vinegar.

Linguine
Calories: 221
Protein: 6.6 g
Fat: 1 g
Sodium: 32 mg
Cholesterol: 0

Tossed Salad
Calories: 29
Protein: 1.7 g
Fat: 0.4 g
Sodium: 8 mg
Cholesterol: 0

13. Vivacious Vegetable Pizza with Asparagus

Serves 2

⅓ cup red bell pepper strips
⅓ cup green bell pepper strips
⅓ cup yellow bell pepper strips
½ cup sliced mushrooms
¼ cup sliced onion
½ cup low-sodium chicken broth
½ cup Classico Mushrooms and Ripe Olives (or other low-fat tomato sauce)

2 teaspoons grated low-fat Parmesan cheese
¾ cup all-purpose flour
⅓ cup wheat germ
¼ teaspoon baking powder
⅓ cup skim milk
1 tablespoon applesauce
1 cup sliced asparagus, cooked

1. Preheat oven to 425°F.
2. "Sauté" vegetables in chicken broth over high heat for 5 to 7 minutes.
3. While the vegetables are cooking, put the tomato sauce in a large cup or small bowl and add the cheese.
4. In a large bowl, combine the flour, wheat germ, and baking powder. Fold in the milk and applesauce and stir until fully blended.
5. Mold the dough into a 7-inch pizza crust and place on a nonstick cookie sheet. Bake for 5 minutes.
6. Add the sauce to the crust, spreading it evenly over the surface. Continue to bake for 14 minutes, or until the crust is golden brown.
7. Cut pizza in half and serve with asparagus on the side.

Note: If you're too lazy to bother with the crust, simply make the sauce and pour it over a toasted whole wheat English muffin or into 2 whole wheat pita breads.

Pizza
Calories: 381
Protein: 19 g
Fat: 3.7 g
Sodium: 153 mg
Cholesterol: 2 mg

Asparagus
Calories: 24
Protein: 2.6 g
Fat: 0.8 g
Sodium: 0
Cholesterol: 0

14. Happy Muscle's Italian Chicken and Rice with Salad and Wheat Germ

Serves 1

¼ cup plus 1 tablespoon wheat germ
½ teaspoon basil
¼ teaspoon oregano
½ teaspoon parsley
⅛ teaspoon garlic powder
⅛ teaspoon paprika
⅛ teaspoon crushed red pepper
1 egg white
1 8-ounce chicken cutlet or 2 4-ounce chicken cutlets
4 ounces low-sodium plain tomato sauce
¼ cup water
1 tablespoon grated low-fat Parmesan cheese
¾ cup cooked white rice, sprinkled with oregano,
    salt (optional), and garlic powder
1 large tomato
¼ head lettuce
Garlic-flavored wine vinegar

1. In a small cup, combine ¼ cup wheat germ, basil, oregano, parsley, garlic powder, paprika, and red pepper. Set aside.

2. In a small dish, beat egg white for 30 seconds.

3. Dip the chicken first in the egg white mixture, then in the wheat germ mixture, and then back again in the egg white mixture until both mixtures are used up—but be sure your final dip is in the wheat.

4. Cook the chicken in a hot nonstick pan over medium heat for 4 minutes on each side.

5. Add the sauce and water to the pan and cook until chicken is done, about 8 minutes. You may add a little water, if necessary.

6. Sprinkle chicken with cheese, cover, and cook for 2 minutes, or until cheese is melted.

7. Serve with rice, sprinkled with any remaining sauce, and tossed salad of lettuce and tomato with wine vinegar dressing. Sprinkle salad with remaining 1 tablespoon wheat germ (optional).

Chicken
Calories: 640
Protein: 94 g
Fat: 12 g
Sodium: 295 mg
Cholesterol: 200 mg

Note: You can cut your calories, fat, protein, and cholesterol in half by halving the size of your chicken breast serving; in other words, start with a 4-ounce chicken cutlet—or, make the recipe as is and use it to serve two!

Rice
Calories: 123
Protein: 2.4 g
Fat: 0.1 g
Sodium: 0
Cholesterol: 0

Large Tossed Salad
Calories: 41
Protein: 2.4 g
Fat: 0.5 g
Sodium: 10 mg
Cholesterol: 0

Wheat Germ (1 tablespoon)
Calories: 38
Protein: 2.7 g
Fat: 1.1 g
Sodium: 0
Cholesterol: 0

15. Feather Kick-Up Fish Stew

Serves 4

1 large onion, diced
1 cup minced celery
½ cup minced carrot
4 new red potatoes, cut into eighths
2 cups water
1 cup low-sodium V-8 juice (or tomato juice)
1 pound sole fillet
1 cup diced broccoli florets
1 cup diced cauliflower florets
½ cup diced carrot
½ teaspoon salt
½ teaspoon onion powder
¼ teaspoon pepper
¼ teaspoon marjoram
¼ teaspoon basil

1. Bring water to a boil in saucepan and add onion, celery, minced carrot, and potatoes. Lower the heat to medium, cover, and cook for 15 minutes.

2. Add all remaining ingredients and continue cooking over low heat for 15 to 20 more minutes, or until potatoes are done. Serve piping hot.

Calories: 398
Protein: 40 g
Fat: 9.4 g
Sodium: 464 mg
Cholesterol: 102 mg

16. Weight-Training Turkey Burgers and Mozzarella Cheese on a Bun with Brussels Sprouts and Tossed Salad

Serves 2

½ pound ground white meat turkey (lean, no fat added)
1 all-purpose potato, cooked, peeled, and mashed
1 egg white
½ cup mild salsa
½ cup low-sodium V-8 juice
1 teaspoon Worcestershire sauce
½ teaspoon onion powder
⅛ teaspoon pepper
⅛ teaspoon chili powder
2 whole wheat burger buns (or rolls)
2 ounces part-skim low-moisture mozzarella cheese
1 cup Brussels sprouts, cooked
½ head lettuce
1 large tomato, quartered
Vinegar and spices to taste for salad (optional)

1. In a large bowl, thoroughly mix turkey, potato, and egg white. Shape the mixture into 2 burgers and set to the side.

2. In a small nonstick frying pan, combine the salsa, V-8, Worcestershire, onion powder, pepper, and chili powder.

3. Place the burgers in the frying pan. They should be covered by the sauce; if not, add some water.

4. Cover and cook over medium heat for 20 minutes, stirring sauce and turning burgers 2 or 3 times.

5. Open the buns and spoon a generous supply of sauce onto both sides of each bun, place a burger on one side of each bun, and spread on a slice of cheese. Close with the other half of the bun.

6. Serve with Brussels sprouts and a tossed salad of lettuce and tomato on the side, sprinkled with vinegar and spices to taste.

Burgers (2)
Calories: 335
Protein: 34 g
Fat: 2.7 g
Sodium: 412 mg
Cholesterol: 70 mg

Mozzarella Cheese
Calories: 79
Protein: 7.8 g
Fat: 4.8 g
Sodium: 150 mg
Cholesterol: 15 mg

Tossed Salad
Calories: 29
Protein: 1.7 g
Fat: 0
Sodium: 8 mg
Cholesterol: 0

Brussels Sprouts
Calories: 30
Protein: 3.5 g
Fat: 0
Sodium: 8 mg
Cholesterol: 0

17. Flounder Patties and Brown Rice with Vegetables

Serves 4

1 pound flounder fillets
½ onion, finely chopped
⅓ cup low-sodium chicken broth
2 teaspoons all-purpose flour
2 egg whites, lightly beaten

2 scallions, chopped
½ cup plain bread crumbs
⅛ teaspoon oregano
⅛ teaspoon basil
2 teaspoons chopped fresh parsley
1 tablespoon dill
½ teaspoon onion powder
⅛ teaspoon pepper
3 cups cooked instant brown rice
4 cups peas and carrots, cooked

1. Place flounder in a microwave dish with 1 inch of water and cook on high for 3 minutes, or broil or steam flounder if you don't have a microwave. Set aside.

2. In a hot roasted frying pan, sauté onion in the broth until soft, then set aside.

3. In a large bowl, combine flour, egg whites, scallions, bread crumbs, oregano, basil, parsley, dill, onion powder, and pepper and mix well.

4. Add the onion and flounder and mix until stiff. Shape into 4 patties.

5. Cook the patties in a nonstick pan for 3 minutes on each side.

6. Combine the brown rice with the peas and carrots and serve with fish.

Fish
Calories: 286
Protein: 38 g
Fat: 9.7 g
Sodium: 373 mg
Cholesterol: 103 mg

Brown Rice and Vegetables
Calories: 178
Protein: 5.6 g
Fat: 0.9 g
Sodium: 72 mg
Cholesterol: 0

18. Vivacious Vegetable Pitas with Blueberries

Serves 1

½ large Spanish onion, minced
¼ red bell pepper, minced
¼ yellow bell pepper, minced
1 small carrot, minced
1 yellow squash, diced
1 small tomato, diced
½ cup diced mushrooms
½ cup low-sodium chicken broth
1 garlic clove, crushed
1 teaspoon Tabasco sauce
¼ teaspoon oregano
¼ teaspoon basil
1 teaspoon parsley
2 whole wheat pita breads
1 cup blueberries

1. "Sauté" vegetables in chicken broth for 5 minutes over high heat, or until slightly soft.
2. Add garlic, Tabasco sauce, oregano, basil, and parsley and cook uncovered over medium heat for 25 minutes.
3. Pour mixture into pita breads and eat while hot. Serve with blueberries.

Note: Pita breads may break up, but it's worth it. Eat with a knife and fork!

Pitas (2)
Calories: 374
Protein: 16 g
Fat: 2.5 g
Sodium: 593 mg
Cholesterol: 0

Blueberries
Calories: 89
Protein: 1.1 g
Fat: 0.6 g
Sodium: 10 mg
Cholesterol: 0

19. All-in-One Lunch: Tofu–Fresh Vegetable Pita Delight

Serves 3

8 ounces firm tofu
⅛ teaspoon crushed red pepper
⅛ teaspoon paprika
½ teaspoon fennel seeds
½ teaspoon curry powder
½ teaspoon chili powder
⅛ teaspoon salt
⅛ teaspoon onion powder
⅛ teaspoon dry mustard
½ cup minced carrot
½ cup minced raw cauliflower florets
½ cup minced Spanish onion
½ cup diced tomato
¼ cup nonfat mayonnaise
3 whole wheat pita breads
3 large lettuce leaves

1. In a large bowl, mash tofu until smooth (or use food processor).
2. Mix in all seasonings. Fold in carrots, cauliflower, onion, and tomato. Add mayonnaise and mix thoroughly.
3. Line pita breads with lettuce leaves and dividing the mixture evenly, fill the pitas to overflowing.

Pita Sandwich
Calories: 245
Protein: 13 g
Fat: 5.2 g
Sodium: 289 mg
Cholesterol: 0

Note: If you use a food processor to dice vegetables, be sure to use the chopping blade or your vegetables will turn to pulpy juice!

20. Chicken and Brown Rice Mushroom Madness

Serves 3

1 pound skinless and boneless chicken breast
1 Spanish onion, thinly sliced
½ cup low-sodium chicken broth
1 red bell pepper, cut into narrow strips
1 green bell pepper, cut into narrow strips
3 plum tomatoes, thinly sliced
6 large mushrooms, thinly sliced
1 teaspoon garlic powder
3 tablespoons chopped parsley
1 bay leaf
2 tablespoons low-sodium soy sauce
¾ cup white wine
1½ cups uncooked instant rice
2 cups water
Sprinkle of paprika

1. Cook chicken in broiler or microwave oven until opaque. Let cool, slice into thin strips, and set aside.
2. In a hot nonstick frying pan, "sauté" onion in chicken broth over high heat until it begins to turn soft, about 5 minutes.

3. Lower heat to medium and add all other ingredients except chicken, rice, water, and paprika. Sauté for 20 minutes, covered, over medium heat.

4. Add the water and heat until near boiling. Add the chicken strips, lower heat, and add the instant rice, stirring rice gently into the mixture. Let simmer for 1 minute, then add more water if mixture seems dry.

5. Remove from heat and wait 5 minutes. Sprinkle with paprika and serve.

Calories: 507
Protein: 56 g
Fat: 6.6 g
Sodium: 464 mg
Cholesterol: 130 mg

21. Strongman's Tangy Tuna

Serves 1

1 10-ounce package frozen chopped spinach (or chopped broccoli)
4 ounces tuna, packed in water
1 small onion, chopped
½ yellow bell pepper, chopped
¼ cup low-sodium chicken broth
1 teaspoon basil
⅛ teaspoon pepper
2 tablespoons balsamic vinegar
2 slices whole wheat bread

1. Cook the spinach or broccoli and squeeze out all excess juice.

2. Drain the tuna and mix well with the spinach or broccoli.

3. In a hot nonstick frying pan, "sauté" the onion and pepper in the broth until slightly soft, about 3 minutes. Add seasonings and vinegar and mix well.

4. Remove from heat and stir into tuna-vegetable mix. Divide evenly and serve on 2 slices of bread.

Calories: 407
Protein: 48 g
Fat: 3.6 g
Sodium: 1431 mg
Cholesterol: 73 mg

22. Kid Gloves Stand-Up Sandwich with Mixed Vegetables

Serves 3

1 15-ounce can kidney beans, rinsed and drained
2 teaspoons plain nonfat yogurt
½ green hot chili pepper, seeded and diced
1 teaspoon garlic powder
1 teaspoon onion powder
1 teaspoon chili powder
3 large romaine lettuce leaves
3 small tomatoes, sliced
6 slices whole wheat bread
3 cups mixed frozen vegetables, cooked

1. Grind the beans in a food processor or place in a large bowl and pummel until completely mashed.
2. Gradually mix in the yogurt, chili pepper, garlic powder, onion powder, and chili powder. Combine thoroughly.
3. Place a lettuce leaf and a sliced tomato on 3 bread slices and coat each with one-third of the mixture.
4. Cover with the other slices of bread. Serve with mixed vegetables on the side.

Sandwich
Calories: 329
Protein: 18 g

Fat: 2.7 g
Sodium: 1 mg
Cholesterol: 1 mg

Mixed Vegetables
Calories: 105
Protein: 5.2 g
Fat: 0.4 g
Sodium: 87 mg
Cholesterol: 0

23. Cutting-Edge Egg White Sandwich and Broccoli

Serves 2

12 egg whites
2 tablespoons nonfat mayonnaise
¼ teaspoon onion powder
¼ teaspoon dry mustard
2 teaspoons dill
Sprinkle of pepper
Sprinkle of paprika
3 large lettuce leaves
4 slices whole wheat bread
2 cups broccoli florets from frozen package or fresh, cooked

1. Hard-boil the eggs about 6 minutes, then rinse under cold water and separate yolks from whites.
2. Discard yolks and finely chop whites. Fold in mayonnaise, onion powder, dry mustard, and dill.
3. Place a lettuce leaf on 2 slices of whole wheat bread. Divide the egg mixture in half and place on the lettuce leaves. Sprinkle with pepper and paprika. Cover with another slice of whole wheat bread for an overflowing sandwich.
4. Serve with broccoli on the side.

Sandwich
Calories: 229
Protein: 24 g
Fat: 1.7 g
Sodium: 530 mg
Cholesterol: 1 mg

Broccoli
Calories: 52
Protein: 6.2 g
Fat: 0.6 g
Sodium: 20 mg
Cholesterol: 0

24. Turkey-Trot Sandwich and Cauliflower

Serves 1

2 tablespoons nonfat mayonnaise
2 teaspoons chopped pickles
2 teaspoons dill
⅛ teaspoon garlic powder
¼ cucumber, thinly sliced
¼ Spanish onion, thinly sliced
½ tomato, thinly sliced
1 large lettuce leaf
2 slices rye bread
2 ounces turkey cutlet
1 cup cauliflower florets, cooked
Sprinkle of paprika

1. Using a small bowl, mix mayonnaise, pickles, dill, and garlic powder.
2. Place the cucumber, onion, tomato, and lettuce on a slice of rye bread. Place turkey on sandwich and finish with other slice of bread.
3. Serve with cauliflower sprinkled with paprika.

Sandwich
Calories: 243
Protein: 19 g
Fat: 1.8 g
Sodium: 356 mg
Cholesterol: 36

Cauliflower
Calories: 25
Protein: 2.6 g
Fat: 0
Sodium: 10 mg
Cholesterol: 0

25. Big-Boy Broiled Pepper and Onion Sandwich with Pineapple

Serves 2

½ Spanish onion, thinly sliced
1 large red bell pepper, sliced into rings
½ large beefsteak tomato, thinly sliced
Sprinkle of garlic powder
Paprika
Sprinkle of salt (optional)
Sprinkle of oregano
¼ teaspoon pepper
1 cup canned black beans, drained
1 tablespoon lemon juice
1 garlic clove
1 ounce grated low-fat Parmesan cheese
1 tablespoon chopped onion
½ teaspoon grated lemon rind
2 romaine lettuce leaves
4 slices pumpernickel bread
4 pineapple slices, or 1 cup pineapple chunks

1. In a preheated broiler, on an aluminum foil–lined broiler pan, spread out the onion, red pepper, and tomato slices. Sprinkle with garlic powder, paprika, salt, oregano, and pepper.

2. Broil for 5 to 6 minutes, or until onion is charred and semisoft.

3. Blend the beans, lemon juice, garlic, cheese, and onion in a food processor or blender until smooth.

4. Place the mixture in a bowl and add lemon rind; mix well.

5. Place lettuce leaves on 2 slices of bread and spread bean mixture evenly.

6. Remove the pepper mixture from the broiler and arrange over the bean mixture. Close the sandwiches with another slice of bread.

7. Serve with pineapple.

Sandwich
Calories: 327
Protein: 17 g
Fat: 1.7 g
Sodium: 425 mg
Cholesterol: 6 mg

Pineapple
Calories: 68
Protein: 0.4 g
Fat: 0.1 g
Sodium: 1 mg
Cholesterol: 0

26. Vitamin-Vixen Vegetable Salmon Sandwich

Serves 2

¼ cup plain nonfat yogurt
½ teaspoon lime juice
⅛ teaspoon cayenne pepper

⅛ teaspoon onion powder
½ teaspoon dill
2 whole wheat pita breads
¼ pickle, diced
¼ cup alfalfa sprouts
¼ cup diced tomato
¼ cup grated carrot
¼ cup diced radishes
½ cup chopped fresh broccoli florets
½ cup chopped fresh cauliflower florets
8 ounces broiled salmon fillet, flaked

1. In a small bowl, mix yogurt, lime juice, and seasonings.
2. Spread the mixture on either side of the pita breads.
3. In a large bowl, combine the pickle, sprouts, tomato, carrot, radishes, broccoli, cauliflower, and salmon.
4. Stuff in pita pockets and top with remaining dressing.

Sandwich
Calories: 186
Protein: 10 g
Fat: 1 g
Sodium: 350 mg
Cholesterol: 1 mg

Salmon
Calories: 206
Protein: 31 g
Fat: 8.3 g
Sodium: 132 mg
Cholesterol: 53 mg

Note: Salmon is calculated separately in case you want to substitute tuna for it, or another lower-fat fish.

27. Bodybuilder's Brown Rice and Chicken Salad

Serves 2

1⅓ cups cooked instant brown rice
2 tablespoons low-sodium chicken broth
1 cup diced skinless chicken breast
⅛ teaspoon onion powder
⅛ teaspoon garlic powder
⅛ teaspoon oregano
⅛ teaspoon basil
⅛ teaspoon paprika
½ celery stalk, diced
½ carrot, grated
¼ cup diced onion
1 large beefsteak tomato, cut into eighths
½ head romaine lettuce
Garlic-flavored wine vinegar
Sprinkle of salt (or onion powder, optional)

    1. In a large mixing bowl, combine rice, chicken broth, chicken, seasonings, and vegetables and mix until fully combined.
    2. Place mixture on top of spread-out leaves of romaine and sprinkle with vinegar and salt.

Calories: 311
Protein: 32 g
Fat: 4 g
Sodium: 94 mg
Cholesterol: 73 mg

28. Luscious Lentil Lift Salad

Serves 2

1 cup brown or red lentils
3 cups water
½ tomato, diced
½ red onion, diced
½ red bell pepper, sliced
½ celery stalk, diced
1 tablespoon dill
¼ teaspoon Mrs. Dash seasoning
½ cup low-fat cottage cheese
½ head romaine lettuce
Sprinkle of paprika
2 slices pumpernickel bread

1. Bring lentils and water to a boil, then reduce heat to medium, cover, and cook for 15 minutes, or until tender but not mushy.
2. Combine tomato, onion, red pepper, celery, dill, seasoning, and cottage cheese, tossing until fully combined.
3. Mix in lentils.
4. Place mixture on a bed of romaine lettuce and sprinkle with paprika. Serve with bread.

Calories: 496
Protein: 36 g
Fat: 2.3 g
Sodium: 459 mg
Cholesterol: 3 mg

29. Top Shape Turkey-Apricot Salad with Wheat Germ

Serves 3

4 ounces canned unsweetened apricots in own juice
¼ cup plain nonfat yogurt
1 tablespoon lime juice
½ tablespoon tarragon
½ tablespoon dill
½ teaspoon dry mustard
¼ teaspoon onion powder
⅛ teaspoon black pepper
¼ teaspoon grated lime peel
2 cups cubed cooked turkey breast
½ unpeeled red apple, diced
½ unpeeled pear, diced
¼ cup raisins
1 head lettuce
6 tablespoons wheat germ (optional)
½ tablespoon chives

1. In a large mixing bowl, combine apricots, yogurt, lime juice, tarragon, dill, mustard, onion powder, pepper, and lime peel. Mix until thoroughly blended.

2. Gradually add turkey, apple, and pear, and mix well.

3. Divide lettuce into 3 parts and arrange on large plates.

4. Divide salad mixture into 3 parts and place each on top of lettuce. Sprinkle with wheat germ, chives, and raisins.

Salad
Calories: 246
Protein: 30 g
Fat: 2.4 g
Sodium: 102 mg
Cholesterol: 71 mg

Wheat Germ (per tablespoon)
Calories: 76
Protein: 5.8 g
Fat: 2.1 g
Sodium: 1 mg
Cholesterol: 0

30. Pyramid Pasta Chicken Salad with Tangerines

Serves 4

8 ounces tricolor pasta swirls, cooked and drained
2 cups cubed cooked skinless chicken breast
⅔ cup diced red bell pepper
½ cup diced cucumber
¼ cup diced red onion
1 cup diced tomato
½ cup sliced mushrooms
½ cup green beans, cooked
½ cup cauliflower florets, cooked
½ cup broccoli florets, cooked
¼ cup white wine
½ teaspoon lemon juice
⅛ teaspoon onion powder (or salt)
⅛ teaspoon oregano
⅛ teaspoon black pepper
1 head lettuce
12 tangerines, separated into sections

1. In a large bowl, mix pasta swirls, chicken, red pepper, cucumber, onion, tomato, mushrooms, beans, cauliflower, and broccoli.
2. Add wine, lemon juice, onion powder, oregano, and black pepper and toss thoroughly.
3. Divide lettuce into 4 parts and arrange salad mixture over lettuce leaves.
4. Serve with tangerines on the side.

Salad
Calories: 434
Protein: 40 g
Fat: 4.7 g
Sodium: 79 mg
Cholesterol: 73 mg

Tangerines (3)
Calories: 66
Protein: 0.9 g
Fat: 0.3 g
Sodium: 2 mg
Cholesterol: 0

31. Self-Esteem Sea Bass and Brown Rice Salad

Serves 2

8 ounces sea bass fillet
1⅓ cups cooked instant brown rice
¼ cup nonfat cottage cheese
2 scallions, diced
½ cucumber, diced
¼ cup Dijon mustard
⅛ teaspoon onion powder
⅛ teaspoon garlic powder
⅛ teaspoon oregano
⅛ teaspoon paprika
⅛ teaspoon black pepper
⅛ teaspoon salt (optional)
½ cup low-sodium V-8 juice
1 lemon
½ head lettuce
2 tomatoes, sliced

1. In a covered microwave dish, cook sea bass in a microwave oven on high in 1 inch of water for 3 minutes, or broil or steam the fish.

2. Using a fork, break the fish into flakelike small pieces and set aside.

3. Place cooked rice in a large mixing bowl and add bass, cottage cheese, scallions, cucumber, mustard, onion powder, garlic powder, oregano, paprika, black pepper, and salt.

4. Mix in V-8 juice, squeeze the lemon into the mix, and blend thoroughly. Chill in the freezer for 15 minutes or refrigerate overnight.

5. Divide the lettuce in half and arrange the leaves on 2 large plates.

6. Distribute the fish evenly over the lettuce leaves. Surround with sliced tomato.

Calories: 359
Protein: 32 g
Fat: 4.2 g
Sodium: 554 mg
Cholesterol: 57 mg

BONUS: SOUPS TO GO WITH SALADS OR SANDWICHES

You could also use these as snacks.

1. Grandma's Old-Fashioned Mushroom Spinach Soup

Serves 6

2 onions, chopped
6 garlic cloves, chopped
1 pound mushrooms, sliced
1 teaspoon sage
⅛ teaspoon pepper
¼ teaspoon onion powder (or salt)
1 8-ounce package frozen whole leaf spinach, thawed
4 cups low-sodium vegetable or chicken broth
1 cup dry red wine
Sprinkle of grated low-fat Parmesan cheese

1. In a nonstick frying pan, sauté the onions, garlic, and mushrooms with the sage, pepper, and onion powder for 7 minutes, or until mushrooms are nearly soft.
2. Add the spinach and cook for 2 more minutes.
3. In a large pot, combine broth and red wine. Add in the spinach mixture, bring to a boil, and reduce heat to medium and cook for 5 minutes.
4. Serve with Parmesan cheese.

Calories: 99
Protein: 5.9 g
Fat: 0.5 g
Sodium: 147 mg
Cholesterol: 2 mg

2. Happy Heart Carrot-Squash Soup

Serves 5

1 small onion, finely chopped
1 garlic clove, finely chopped
1 small tomato, diced
½ teaspoon oregano
½ teaspoon onion powder (or salt)
¼ teaspoon pepper
2 cups peeled sliced carrots
1 cup sliced yellow squash
2½ cups low-sodium beef broth
⅓ cup nonfat dry milk
½ teaspoon apple juice concentrate

1. In a large nonstick frying pan, sauté the onion, garlic, tomato, oregano, onion powder, and pepper for 5 minutes, then set aside.

2. Steam the carrots and squash until tender.

3. Using a blender or food processor, mix the carrots and squash, adding broth as you go until smooth. Add dry milk and apple juice concentrate and continue to blend until a smooth puree is formed.

4. Pour puree into the onion-garlic mixture (if it fits in the frying pan, otherwise transfer both mixtures to a large pot). Pour in remaining beef broth and mix well. Cook until steaming hot.

Calories: 78
Protein: 4.7 g
Fat: 0
Sodium: 144 mg
Cholesterol: 1 mg

3. Boom-Boom Black Bean Soup

Serves 8

3 cups canned black beans
4 cups low-sodium vegetable or chicken broth
1 large new red potato, diced
½ cup shredded carrots
½ cup low-sodium V-8 juice
2 tablespoons low-sodium soy sauce
1 teaspoon dill
1 teaspoon parsley
1 teaspoon basil
½ teaspoon onion powder
¼ teaspoon pepper

1. In a large pot, mix all ingredients, cover, and cook over medium heat for 45 minutes.

2. Remove the solid material from the soup using a strainer and place in food processor or blender. Mix until a smooth puree.

3. Return puree to soup pot, blend well, and cook for 3 minutes, or until piping hot.

Calories: 120
Protein: 7.8 g
Fat: 0.5 g
Sodium: 212 mg
Cholesterol: 0

4. Rousing Russian Potato Soup

Serves 5

1 cup low-sodium chicken broth
1 16-ounce can crushed tomatoes
1 8-ounce can low-sodium V-8 juice

6 large new potatoes, peeled
1 celery stalk, finely chopped
1 large carrot, shredded
1 large onion, diced
1 cup shredded cabbage
1 tablespoon dry mustard
1 tablespoon apple juice concentrate
1 tablespoon parsley
1 tablespoon dill
2 to 3 cups water (2 if eating right away, 3 if storing overnight)

1. Combine all ingredients and place in a pressure cooker for 7 minutes, or bring to a boil, cover, and cook over medium-low heat for 45 minutes.
2. Serve piping hot.

Calories: 193
Protein: 6 g
Fat: 1 g
Sodium: 182 mg
Cholesterol: 0

5. Beat-the-Hunger Broccoli-Cauliflower-Carrot Soup

Serves 6

2 cups chopped broccoli
½ cup chopped cauliflower
½ cup diced carrots
1 small onion, finely chopped
1 garlic clove, minced
½ teaspoon basil
½ teaspoon oregano
½ teaspoon onion powder (or salt)
⅛ teaspoon pepper
1 tablespoon wine vinegar
2 cups low-sodium chicken broth
⅓ cup nonfat dry milk

1. Steam broccoli, cauliflower, and carrots until nearly soft, then set aside to cool.

2. Combine the onion, garlic, basil, oregano, onion powder, pepper, vinegar, and broth in a soup pot and cook over moderate heat until onions are tender.

3. Place broccoli-cauliflower-carrot mixture in the food processor and blend until pureed. Add dry milk to food processed mixture and blend until smooth.

4. Pour the milk mixture into the soup pot and heat until nearly boiling. Serve piping hot.

Calories: 55
Protein: 4.8 g
Fat: 0
Sodium: 91 mg
Cholesterol: 1 mg

6. Accent on Asparagus Pea Soup

Serves 5

3 cups chopped fresh asparagus
1 small onion, diced
½ cup shredded carrot
¼ cup diced celery
⅓ cup white wine
¼ teaspoon dill
⅛ teaspoon black pepper
½ teaspoon garlic powder
¼ cup water
⅔ cup frozen peas, cooked
2 cups low-sodium chicken broth
¼ cup nonfat dry milk
½ lemon, squeezed for juice

1. Steam asparagus for about 6 minutes, then set aside.
2. Place onion, carrot, celery, wine, dill, pepper, and garlic

powder in a nonstick skillet. Add water and sauté over high heat until onion is tender, about 5 minutes.

3. Place the asparagus and peas in a food processor or blender and mix until pureed, using the chicken broth to get the right consistency. Add powdered milk to the food processed mixture and blend until uniform.

4. Remove mixture from food processor and place in a soup pot. Add onion-carrot mixture and stir until thoroughly blended.

5. Add remaining chicken broth and lemon juice and bring to near boil. Serve piping hot.

Note: The lemon is everything. It really pulls it all together.

Calories: 90
Protein: 7.2 g
Fat: 0.3 g
Sodium: 196 mg
Cholesterol: 1 mg

7. Gut Buster Gazpacho Soup

Serves 4

8 plum tomatoes, diced
1 zucchini, steamed and diced
1 red bell pepper, chopped
1 large Spanish onion, chopped
¼ cup chopped spinach, cooked
⅛ teaspoon garlic powder
⅛ teaspoon chili powder
⅛ teaspoon crushed red pepper
⅛ teaspoon oregano
⅛ teaspoon basil
⅛ teaspoon black pepper
⅛ teaspoon salt
1 cup low-sodium V-8 juice

1. Combine all ingredients and refrigerate for 10 to 14 hours. Place mixture in a sealed container so ingredients are airtight and spices can mix well.

2. Serve cold.

Calories: 93
Protein: 4.9 g
Fat: 0.8 g
Sodium: 50 mg
Cholesterol: 0

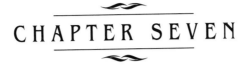

CHAPTER SEVEN

DINNER MENUS FOR A MONTH

Dinner! Some of us live for it. I'm one of those people. In the following pages you will find ten dinners that are quick and easy and twenty-one that take a little preparation.

UNDERSTANDING THE NUTRITIONAL INFORMATION

Following each recipe are one or more nutritional analyses listing the calorie content plus protein, fat, sodium, and carbohydrate found in the food. The calculations are *per serving* unless otherwise indicated. For example, in a recipe serving four persons, the analysis will be for one serving. For a recipe yielding six blintzes, two blintzes constituting a serving, the analysis will be for two blintzes.

You will note that when fruit or a vegetable is added as a side dish, the calculations are shown separately—one analysis for the main dish and one for the side dish—so that you have detailed information on the food values of the specific foods you are eating. Also, if you are using the recipes to make up your own meal plans, you might want to eliminate or substitute the side dish.

Protein and fat measures are shown in grams (g); sodium and carbohydrate contents are given in milligrams (mg). Refer to Chapter 3 for guidelines on using these figures. Bear in mind, however, that the meal plans in Chapter 9 count everything for you—these analyses are for your information in case you want to make your own daily meal plans.

When an alternative ingredient appears in parentheses, this means the substitute has not been included in the analysis. For example, "1 teaspoon garlic powder (or salt)" means that the analysis includes garlic powder but not salt (which would yield a higher sodium content).

When recipes include wheat germ or canola oil, the analysis for these items is usually kept separate. I've added these items in the recipe to meet the fat requirements in the meal plans, but if you are developing your own meal plans, you might want to omit these items and obtain your fat minimum in another way. On the rare occasions when it is included in the recipe, it is because I feel it is absolutely necessary to the taste of the recipe.

A NOTE ABOUT THE RECIPES

Where nonstick cookware is involved, it is assumed that you have lightly coated the cookware with a vegetable oil cooking spray, like Pam.

When 1 percent dairy products are used, feel free to substitute nonfat products. I use the 1 percent items when I feel you need that bit of fat to fulfill a healthy daily fat requirement. (The minimum fat you should get is 10 percent of total caloric intake.)

Feel free to substitute the fruit or vegetable on the side with any other fruit or vegetable, or eliminate the item at the meal and eat it any other time of the day. You may replace the side-dish vegetable suggestions with any other vegetables from the equivalent lists in Chapter 3. In other words, you must replace unlimited complex carbohydrate vegetables with unlimited and limited with limited. Also feel free to cut the serving size in half if you feel it is too much for you.

Fruits and vegetables in the ingredients lists are medium size unless otherwise indicated. Herbs and spices are dried unless fresh is indicated. When I call for cooked vegetables and don't specify how to cook them, you can cook them any way you please as long as it's a nonfat method. Also, you can use either fresh or frozen vegetables.

If you're making up your own meal plans, feel free to eliminate the canola oil. (I've calculated it separately.) I've used the oil on occasion to fulfill the daily fat requirement for my meal plans.

QUICK AND EASY MEALS

1. Microwave Vegetable-Flounder Stew with White Rice

Serves 1

6 ounces flounder fillet
1 red bell pepper, cut into strips
1 onion, sliced
10 fresh mushrooms, sliced
1 zucchini, sliced (or yellow summer squash)
1 tomato, cubed
¼ teaspoon oregano
½ teaspoon garlic powder
⅛ teaspoon paprika
⅛ teaspoon pepper
⅛ teaspoon salt (optional)
½ cup white wine
2½ cups water
½ cup uncooked instant white rice

1. Place fish and vegetables in a large microwave dish.

2. Sprinkle with seasonings and add wine. Pour in water. Cover and cook in microwave oven on high for 15 minutes.

3. Add rice, mix, and cover; let stand for 10 minutes.

Note: Add water as necessary, to your liking. Also note that the rice when cooked swells to about 1 cup, so this is quite a hearty meal. I eat this in two or three sittings over an hour's time.

Also, you can cook this in a 350°F. oven for 35 minutes instead.

Calories: 473
Protein: 37 g
Fat: 2.3 g
Sodium: 284 mg
Cholesterol: 103 mg

2. Microwave Dill-Sole Stew with Brown Rice

Serves 1

6 ounces sole fillet
1 green bell pepper, sliced
1 red bell pepper, sliced
2 onions, sliced
3 tomatoes, cut into eighths
⅛ teaspoon celery seed
2 teaspoons dill
½ teaspoon parsley
⅛ teaspoon light salt
⅛ teaspoon paprika
½ teaspoon garlic powder
1 tablespoon white wine
3 cups water
½ cup uncooked instant brown rice

1. Place fish and vegetables in a microwave dish.

2. Sprinkle with seasonings and add wine. Pour in water, cover, and cook in microwave oven on high for 15 minutes.

3. Add rice, mix, and cover; let stand for 10 minutes. If water has evaporated, add 3/4 cup water as needed.

Calories: 655
Protein: 41 g
Fat: 4.1 g
Sodium: 255 mg
Cholesterol: 103 mg

3. Tossed Tofu Dinner in a Salad with Pita Bread and Grapefruit

Serves 2

½ small head lettuce, roughly chopped
2 large tomatoes, roughly chopped
4 fresh mushrooms, sliced
1 onion, thinly sliced
1 cucumber, diced
1 red bell pepper, diced
½ cup peas (frozen), cooked
½ lemon
6 ounces tofu, cubed
⅛ teaspoon paprika
⅛ teaspoon oregano
⅛ teaspoon rosemary
⅛ teaspoon salt
2 whole wheat pita breads
1 grapefruit, halved

1. Place lettuce in a large bowl and add tomatoes, mushrooms, onion, cucumber, red pepper, and peas. Toss.

2. Squeeze the juice from the lemon and toss with salad.

3. Add tofu and seasonings and toss again.

4. Stuff part of the salad into the pitas and eat the rest on the side, with grapefruit.

Salad
Calories: 352
Protein: 23 g
Fat: 6 g
Sodium: 529 mg
Cholesterol: 0

Whole Wheat Pita
Calories: 106
Protein: 4 g
Fat: 0.6 g
Sodium: 215 mg
Cholesterol: 0

1/2 Grapefruit
Calories: 32
Protein: 0.6 g
Fat: 0
Sodium: 1 mg
Cholesterol: 0

4. Broiled Red Snapper, Red Peppers, and Onions with Corn on the Cob

Serves 1

8 ounces red snapper fillet (or talapia)
1 large red bell pepper, sliced
1 green bell pepper, sliced
1 large onion, sliced
1 large tomato, sliced

Generous sprinkle of oregano, paprika, garlic powder, pepper, and optional salt
1 medium ear corn on the cob

1. Line a broiler pan with aluminum foil. Do not cut slits to drain.

2. Place red snapper in the center of the pan and arrange peppers, onion, and tomato around the fish, covering the whole pan and, if necessary, placing some vegetables on top of each other and the fish. (I like to put some onion rings over the tomatoes.) Sprinkle thoroughly with seasonings.

3. Broil about 4 inches from the heat for 6 to 8 minutes, or until fish flakes. Some of the vegetables will be charred—all the better!

4. Serve with corn on the cob.

Fish
Calories: 316
Protein: 49 g
Fat: 2.7 g
Sodium: 293 mg
Cholesterol: 80 mg

Corn on the Cob
Calories: 100
Protein: 3.3 g
Fat: 1 g
Sodium: 1 mg
Cholesterol: 0

5. Marinated Chicken and Orzo

Serves 4

¼ cup low-sodium soy sauce
1½ tablespoons cornstarch
¼ cup water
8 ounces boneless and skinless chicken breasts, cut into strips
½ cup low-sodium chicken broth
1 green bell pepper, chopped
2 red bell peppers, chopped
1 large onion, chopped
¼ cup chopped fresh parsley
½ cup tomato sauce
1 cup water
2⅔ cups cooked orzo

1. Place soy sauce in bowl and add cornstarch; mix until thoroughly blended, adding water as you mix. Add chicken strips and set aside to marinate for 30 minutes.

2. Heat broth in large nonstick skillet over high heat and add peppers, onion, and parsley. "Sauté" over high heat for 7 minutes, or until onion is nearly soft, stirring often. (Note: If liquid evaporates, add ¼ cup water.)

3. Add tomato sauce and water. Pour chicken into pepper mixture and cook over low heat for 15 minutes, or until chicken is cooked through.

4. Serve over orzo, allowing ⅔ cup orzo per person.

Calories: 443
Protein: 45 g
Fat: 4.9 g
Sodium: 572 mg
Cholesterol: 98 mg

6. Broiled Flounder and Tomatoes, Mushrooms, and Onions with Broccoli and Fried Brown Rice

Serves 1

8 ounces flounder fillet
1 large tomato, sliced
1 large red pepper, cut into rings
12 fresh mushrooms, sliced
1 large onion, sliced
Generous sprinkling of dill, oregano, paprika, pepper, and
   optional salt
1 teaspoon canola oil (optional)
⅔ cup cooked instant brown rice
1 cup broccoli florets, cooked

1. Line a broiler pan with aluminum foil. Do not cut slits to drain.
2. Place flounder in the center of the pan and arrange vegetables around the fish, overlapping and covering fish if necessary. Sprinkle thoroughly with seasonings.
3. Broil about 4 inches from the heat for 6 minutes, or until fish flakes. Some of the vegetables will be charred. All the better!
4. Coat a nonstick pan with oil and "fry" the brown rice for 1 minute, stirring constantly.
5. Serve with broccoli and brown rice.

Note: You can eliminate the "frying" of the rice and save the fat grams for something else, if you're making your own meal plans.

Fish
Calories: 379
Protein: 45 g
Fat: 3.3 g
Sodium: 276 mg
Cholesterol: 137 mg

Broccoli
Calories: 52
Protein: 6.2 g
Fat: 0.6 g
Sodium: 20 mg
Cholesterol: 0

Brown Rice
Calories: 119
Protein: 2.5 g
Fat: 0.6 g
Sodium: 2 mg
Cholesterol: 0

Canola Oil
Calories: 38
Protein: 0
Fat: 4.2 g
Sodium: 0
Cholesterol: 0

7. Broiled Sole and the Works with Capri Vegetables

Serves 1

8 ounces sole fillet
2 large tomatoes
12 fresh mushrooms, sliced
1 large red onion, sliced
2 large red bell peppers, sliced
Generous sprinkling of dill, oregano, paprika, pepper, garlic
    powder, crushed red pepper (see Note), and optional salt
1 cup Capri frozen vegetables, cooked (see Note)

1. Line a broiler pan with aluminum foil. Do not cut slits to drain.

2. Place sole in the center of the pan and scatter vegetables around the fish, covering the whole pan and, if necessary, placing some of the vegetables on top of each other and the fish. Sprinkle thoroughly with seasonings.

3. Broil about 4 inches from the heat for 6 to 8 minutes, or until fish flakes. Some of the vegetables will be charred. All the better!

4. Serve with vegetables.

Note: Don't be too generous with the crushed red pepper.

I selected the Capri vegetables because it is an interesting mix. You can substitute any other vegetable mixture, only be sure no fat has been added.

Fish
Calories: 405
Protein: 47 g
Fat: 3.6 g
Sodium: 288 mg
Cholesterol: 137 mg

Vegetables
Calories: 105
Protein: 5.2 g
Fat: 0.4 g
Sodium: 87 g
Cholesterol: 0

8. Broiled Chicken Breast with Carrots and White Rice

Serves 1

8 ounces skinless chicken breast, bone in
Generous sprinkle of oregano, paprika, onion powder, pepper,
   and optional salt
1 cup sliced carrots, cooked
⅔ cup cooked instant white rice

1. Line a broiler pan with aluminum foil and slit to drain.
2. Place the chicken in the pan and sprinkle with seasonings on both sides.
3. Broil for 10 minutes, then turn over and broil another 10 minutes, or until cooked through.
4. Serve with carrots and rice sprinkled with seasonings to taste.

Note: Since mushrooms and tomatoes are free, you may want to slice some and add them to the broiler pan 8 minutes before chicken is done.

Chicken
Calories: 286
Protein: 54 g
Fat: 5.9 g
Sodium: 232 mg
Cholesterol: 146 mg

Carrots
Calories: 47
Protein: 1.4 g
Fat: 0.2 g
Sodium: 50 mg
Cholesterol: 0

White Rice
Calories: 109
Protein: 2 g
Fat: 0.1 g
Sodium: 0
Cholesterol: 0

9. Stir-Fried Vegetables and Brown Rice with Turkey Breast

Serves 1

1 16-ounce package frozen stir-fried vegetables, cooked
1 teaspoon canola oil (optional)
½ cup cooked turkey breast, cubed
⅛ teaspoon oregano
⅛ teaspoon dill
⅛ teaspoon salt
⅔ cup cooked instant brown rice
1 celery stalk, minced
1 onion, chopped

1. Stir-fry the vegetables in the oil until lightly browned (see Note).
2. Place the hot vegetables in a large bowl and add the cubed turkey breast. Stir in the oregano, dill, and salt and toss thoroughly.
3. Add the brown rice, celery, and onion and toss well.

Note: You can stir-fry the vegetables "as is," with no oil, in a nonstick pan and save the fat grams for other foods if you're making your own meal plans. I needed the fat grams for my daily requirement in my meal plans.

Vegetables and Rice
Calories: 411
Protein: 44 g
Fat: 4.1 g
Sodium: 469 mg
Cholesterol: 70 mg

Canola Oil
Calories: 38
Protein: 0
Fat: 4.2 g
Sodium: 0
Cholesterol: 0

10. Pasta with Vegetables and Springtime Salad

Serves 1

1 cup cooked linguine
1 cup broccoli and cauliflower mix (from frozen package), cooked
½ cup Healthy Choice Garlic and Herbs Pasta Sauce (or other low-fat tomato sauce)
½ head romaine lettuce
1 large tomato, cut into eighths
2 tablespoons balsamic vinegar

1. Place pasta in a saucepan and mix in broccoli and cauliflower. Add sauce and mix. Cook over medium heat for 1 minute, or until hot; add a little water if necessary to keep from sticking to pan.
2. Chop lettuce and put in bowl with tomatoes.
3. Toss salad with balsamic vinegar and serve with pasta mix.

Note: I've kept the vegetable analysis separate because you might want to experiment with different vegetables.

Pasta
Calories: 270
Protein: 9.3 g
Fat: 2.1 g
Sodium: 37 mg
Cholesterol: 0

Broccoli and Cauliflower
Calories: 39
Protein: 4.2 g
Fat: 0.4 g
Sodium: 20 mg
Cholesterol: 0

Salad
Calories: 45
Protein: 2.2 g
Fat: 0.5 g
Sodium: 9 mg
Cholesterol: 0

Bonus Rice and Beans (My Favorite Quickie)

Serves 1

½ cup canned small red beans (calculations for Goya brand)
1 cup cooked instant white rice
Sprinkle of onion powder
Sprinkle of garlic powder
Sprinkle of chili powder
Sprinkle of curry powder

1. Heat beans in their own juice and remove from heat.

2. Drain beans and combine with rice. Sprinkle with spices and stir thoroughly. (You may choose to keep the liquid—it makes the dish taste even better.)

3. Serve hot. (I sometimes double the beans.)

Note: You can add ½ chopped onion for flavor.

Beans
Calories: 90
Protein: 7 g
Fat: 0.1 g
Sodium: 380 mg
Cholesterol: 0

Rice
Calories: 180
Protein: 4 g
Fat: 0
Sodium: 0.5 mg
Cholesterol: 0

DINNERS THAT TAKE A LITTLE LONGER

11. Joyce's Security Blanket Chicken Soup and Rice

Serves 4

4 skinless whole chicken breasts with bone
7 carrots, cut in half
2 parsnips, cut in half
4 parsley sprigs
7 onions, chopped
8 celery stalks, cut in half
2 teaspoons salt (or to taste)
½ teaspoon pepper
12 cups water
2 cups uncooked instant white rice

1. Place the first 8 ingredients in an 8-quart pot and add water. The water should not rise higher than about 2 inches from the top of the pot; use less if necessary.

2. Cover and bring to a hearty boil. Remove brown foam that rises to the surface.

3. Cover and cook on medium-low heat for 30 minutes, or until vegetables are tender. Turn off flame. (I sometimes deliberately overcook for 45 minutes and let the chicken break up into the soup.)

4. Add the rice to soup. Let stand for 15 minutes. Or you may instead simply cook rice separately and serve ¾ cup with 2 cups of soup per serving.

Note: I often double the amount of rice (using the first method—putting it in the soup). Although this adds 200 calories per serving, it's worth it—it really makes the soup thick!

Calories: 755
Protein: 81 g
Fat: 10 g
Sodium: 727 mg
Cholesterol: 195 mg

12. Martha's Russian Cheese Blintzes and Broccoli

Serves 2; makes 6 blintzes, 3 blintzes per serving

½ cup all-purpose flour
Pinch of salt
4 egg whites and 1 egg yolk
1 tablespoon applesauce
1 cup 1% milk
1½ cups low-fat cottage cheese
2 cups broccoli florets, cooked

1. Mix flour and salt in medium bowl, making a well in the middle.

2. Add the egg whites and yolk and stir the applesauce into the well.

3. Add half the milk and, with a wooden spoon, gradually stir the flour into the center mixture until fully blended.

4. Add the rest of the milk and mix until smooth.

5. Use a ⅓-cup measure to spoon out batter into a 10-inch nonstick skillet. Rolling batter around in the pan until evenly distributed, cook blintze until slightly browned, then turn and cook until brown on second side.

6. Repeat for remaining blintzes. You will have to respray with vegetable oil after each 2 blintzes.

7. Place a little cottage cheese at the edge of each blintze and roll up. Place blintzes in a nonstick frying pan, cover, and heat until cottage cheese begins to melt.

8. Serve with broccoli on the side.

Blintzes (3)
Calories: 370
Protein: 38 g
Fat: 6.1 g
Sodium: 944 mg
Cholesterol: 146 mg

Broccoli
Calories: 48
Protein: 5.4 g
Fat: 0.5 g
Sodium: 23 mg
Cholesterol: 0

13. Poppy Joe's Sole Paella

Serves 4

1 large onion, chopped
4 cups low-sodium beef broth
6 garlic cloves, minced
1 red bell pepper, diced
4 cups cooked instant brown rice
4 tomatoes, chopped
1 pound sole fillets, cooked
Pinch of saffron
⅛ teaspoon oregano
⅛ teaspoon pepper
⅛ teaspoon onion powder
2 teaspoons salt (optional)
1 cup peas, cooked

1. In a large nonstick frying pan, "sauté" onion in ¼ cup broth until nearly soft, about 5 minutes.

2. Add garlic, red pepper, and rice and cook for 1 minute, stirring continually.

3. Add the rest of the broth, tomatoes, fish, saffron, oregano, pepper, onion powder, and salt. Bring to a boil, lower heat, and simmer for 5 minutes.

4. Stir in peas and cook for 10 minutes, stirring every 4 minutes.

5. Serve piping hot.

Calories: 501
Protein: 45 g
Fat: 11 g
Sodium: 612 mg
Cholesterol: 102 mg

14. Cheeky Chicken and Brown Rice Pilaf
with Green Beans and Carrots

Serves 4

1 large onion
1 cup grated carrots
½ cup diced red bell pepper
¼ cup low-sodium chicken broth
2 large oranges, grated, rind included
¼ cup raisins
¼ teaspoon turmeric
2⅔ cups uncooked instant brown rice
2½ cups hot water
1½ cups diced cooked chicken breast
Sprinkle of paprika
2 cups green beans, cooked
2 cups sliced carrots, cooked

1. Sauté the onion, grated carrots, and red pepper in the broth for 5 minutes, or until onion is nearly tender.
2. Add the grated orange, raisins, and turmeric and mix thoroughly. Cook for 1 minute.
3. Add the brown rice, mix thoroughly, stir in hot water, and bring to a boil. Cover and simmer for 12 minutes.
4. Add the chicken and cook for 3 minutes.
5. Sprinkle with paprika and serve with green beans and carrots on the side.

Chicken and Rice
Calories: 741
Protein: 39 g
Fat: 5.8 g
Sodium: 103 mg
Cholesterol: 73 mg

Green Beans and Carrots
Calories: 48
Protein: 2.3 g
Fat: 0
Sodium: 29 mg
Cholesterol: 0

15. Sporty Stuffed Red Peppers with Brussels Sprouts

Serves 4

1 large onion, chopped
¼ cup low-sodium chicken broth
½ cup chopped mushrooms
½ cup chopped celery
½ cup chopped zucchini
3 large tomatoes, chopped
½ teaspoon garlic powder
2 teaspoons oregano
2 tablespoons chopped parsley
1 teaspoon basil
⅛ teaspoon pepper
1 teaspoon salt
3 cups cooked instant brown rice
1 cup water
4 large red bell peppers, halved lengthwise
Sprinkle of grated nonfat Parmesan cheese
4 cups Brussels sprouts, cooked

    1. Preheat oven to 400°F.
    2. In a large nonstick frying pan, "sauté" onion in chicken broth for 5 minutes, or until the onion turns slightly soft.
    3. Add the mushrooms, celery, and zucchini. Mix thoroughly and cook for 3 minutes.
    4. Add the tomatoes, garlic powder, oregano, parsley, basil, pepper, salt, and rice. Add water and mix thoroughly. If mixture is dry, add additional water.

5. Stuff peppers and place in nonstick baking dish. Cover and bake for 30 minutes. (Note: If you have leftover mixture you may stuff some extra peppers.)

6. Sprinkle peppers with cheese and serve with Brussels sprouts on the side.

Peppers (2)
Calories: 194
Protein: 6.2 g
Fat: 1.2 g
Sodium: 44 mg
Cholesterol: 1 mg

Brussels Sprouts
Calories: 60
Protein: 7 g
Fat: 0.6 g
Sodium: 17 mg
Cholesterol: 0

16. Racy Fried Rice and Chicken with Zucchini

Serves 4

½ teaspoon canola oil
½ cup diced red bell pepper
¼ cup sliced mushrooms
3 tablespoons frozen peas, thawed
¾ cup diced cooked chicken breast
¼ cup diced red onion
¼ cup grated carrots
¼ cup diced pineapple
1 tablespoon chopped fresh cilantro
⅛ teaspoon celery seed
3½ cups cooked instant brown rice
¼ cup low-sodium chicken broth
¼ cup low-sodium soy sauce
4 cups chopped zucchini, cooked

1. Heat oil in a large nonstick frying pan until hot and add red pepper, mushrooms, peas, chicken, onion, carrots, pineapple, cilantro, and celery seed. Mix thoroughly and sauté for 5 minutes, or until onion is nearly soft.

2. Add rice, chicken broth, and soy sauce and mix thoroughly. Stirring continually, cook over medium heat until most of the liquid evaporates.

3. Serve with zucchini on the side.

Rice and Chicken
Calories: 271
Protein: 19 g
Fat: 3 g
Sodium: 564 mg
Cholesterol: 37 mg

Zucchini
Calories: 28
Protein: 1.8 g
Fat: 0.2 g
Sodium: 2 mg
Cholesterol: 0

17. Hot Flounder Chili Fillets with Spinach

Serves 4

1 16-ounce can whole tomatoes
1 16-ounce can kidney beans, rinsed and drained
2 teaspoons chili powder
1 teaspoon curry powder
1 onion, finely chopped
½ cup water
4 6-ounce flounder fillets
Sprinkle of oregano, garlic powder, and crushed red pepper
2 cups spinach, cooked

1. Mix tomatoes and beans in a bowl, add in chili and curry powder, and set aside.

2. "Sauté" onion in nonstick skillet over medium-high heat with water for 5 minutes, or until onion is semisoft. Stir frequently.

3. Add onion to tomato-bean mix and set aside.

4. Sprinkle each fillet on both sides with oregano, garlic powder, and a touch of crushed red pepper. Cook each side for 1 minute over medium heat in a nonstick skillet.

5. Pour tomato-bean mixture over the fillets, cover, and cook for 5 to 6 minutes, or until fish flakes when you pierce it with fork.

6. Serve with spinach on the side.

Fish
Calories: 523
Protein: 62 g
Fat: 15 g
Sodium: 600 mg
Cholesterol: 153 mg

Spinach
Calories: 23
Protein: 3 g
Fat: 0.3 g
Sodium: 52 mg
Cholesterol: 0

18. Titanium Woman's Turkey Cutlets and Linguine with Cucumbers and Tomatoes

Serves 4

4 8-ounce turkey breast cutlets
2 tablespoons Dijon mustard
Sprinkle of oregano, rosemary, tarragon, garlic powder, pepper, and paprika

1 onion, minced
1½ cups low-sodium chicken broth
½ cup dry white wine
2⅔ cups cooked linguine
4 tomatoes, thinly sliced
4 cucumbers, thinly sliced
Wine vinegar
Sprinkle of salt (optional)

1. Rinse cutlets and blot dry with a paper towel. Coat on both sides with mustard.

2. Sprinkle cutlets with oregano, rosemary, tarragon, garlic powder, pepper, and paprika and set aside.

3. In a nonstick frying pan, "sauté" onion in ½ cup of the broth until nearly soft, about 5 minutes.

4. Add cutlets to pan, spooning the onion on top of the cutlets. Cook for 2 minutes on each side over medium heat.

5. Add the rest of the broth and the wine. Cover and simmer for 10 minutes, or until chicken is cooked through.

6. Serve with linguine, using the wine–chicken broth juice as a sauce.

7. Arrange the tomatoes and cucumbers on a plate and sprinkle with vinegar and salt.

Turkey and Linguine
Calories: 406
Protein: 59 g
Fat: 4.5 g
Sodium: 245 mg
Cholesterol: 141 mg

Cucumber and Tomatoes
Calories: 47
Protein: 2.1 g
Fat: 0.5 g
Sodium: 11 mg
Cholesterol: 0

19. Amazing Mushroom Tofu Burgers
with Tomato and Onion

Serves 4

12 ounces firm tofu
3 tablespoons grated carrot
2 tablespoons minced onion
¼ cup chopped mushrooms
1 tablespoon Italian bread crumbs
½ teaspoon salt
2 egg whites
1 cup low-sodium chicken broth
1 large beefsteak tomato, sliced
1 large red onion, sliced

1. Cut tofu into small squares and place in large bowl.
2. Mash tofu and mix in carrot, onion, mushrooms, bread crumbs, and salt. Add egg whites and mix thoroughly. Shape into 4 burgers.
3. In a small skillet, heat chicken broth to boiling and add tofu burgers. Cook for 2 minutes on each side. (Or place burgers in a hot nonstick skillet and fry over medium-high heat for 2 minutes on each side.)
4. Remove from skillet and place burgers on top of tomato slices. Top with a slice of red onion.

Note: You may use the leftover broth as a soup—it will have delicious tofu morsels in it.

Burgers
Calories: 101
Protein: 9.9 g
Fat: 4 g
Sodium: 230 mg
Cholesterol: 0

Tomato and Onion
Calories: 69
Protein: 2.7 g
Fat: 0.5 g
Sodium: 7 mg
Cholesterol: 0

20. Sweet-and-Sour Tofu Mini-Burgers with Brown Rice and Broccoli

Serves 2

1 egg
12 ounces soft tofu
½ cup plain bread crumbs
3 tablespoons parsley
⅛ teaspoon pepper
2 tablespoons apple juice concentrate
½ lemon, squeezed for juice
1⅓ cups cooked instant brown rice
2 cups broccoli florets, cooked

1. Lightly beat egg and set aside.
2. Squeeze tofu in a paper towel to remove excess water. Place in a large bowl and add bread crumbs, beaten egg, parsley, pepper, apple juice concentrate, and lemon juice.
3. Mix thoroughly and shape into 6 mini-burgers.
4. Cook burgers in a large nonstick skillet for about 5 minutes over medium-high heat, turning 2 or 3 times so that burgers are slightly browned.
5. Serve on a bed of brown rice, with broccoli on the side.

Mini-Burgers (3)
Calories: 611
Protein: 29 g
Fat: 14 g
Sodium: 600 mg
Cholesterol: 136 mg

Broccoli
Calories: 52
Protein: 6.2 g
Fat: 0.6 g
Sodium: 20 mg
Cholesterol: 0

Brown Rice
Calories: 119
Protein: 2.5 g
Fat: 0.6 g
Sodium: 2 mg
Cholesterol: 0

21. Protein-Power Tofu-Potatoes and Zucchini

Serves 4

4 large baking potatoes
1 onion, minced
¼ cup minced green bell pepper
½ cup low-sodium chicken broth
12 ounces firm tofu, cut into small squares
¼ teaspoon salt
⅛ teaspoon pepper
⅛ teaspoon oregano
⅛ teaspoon garlic powder
¼ cup grated nonfat Parmesan cheese
Sprinkle of paprika
2 cups sliced zucchini, cooked

1. Preheat oven to 350°F. (or use a microwave oven).
2. Bake potatoes about 30 minutes (or 8 minutes on high in microwave).
3. Cut potatoes in half and remove a good deal of the insides. Place the pulp in a mixing bowl and set aside.

4. In nonstick frying pan, "sauté" onion and green pepper over high heat in chicken broth for 5 minutes, or until slightly soft.

5. Add onion-pepper combination to potato pulp and mix well. Add tofu, salt, pepper, oregano, and garlic powder and mix well, mashing the tofu thoroughly.

6. Stuff mixture back into the potato shells and sprinkle with cheese and paprika.

7. Bake for 7 minutes (or 2 minutes on high in microwave), or until heated through.

8. Serve with zucchini on the side.

Potato
Calories: 306
Protein: 15 g
Fat: 4 g
Sodium: 132 mg
Cholesterol: 5 mg

Zucchini
Calories: 12
Protein: 1 g
Fat: 0
Sodium: 1 mg
Cholesterol: 0

22. Leg-Curl Eggplant Lasagne with Carrots, Asparagus, and Salad

Serves 4

8 ounces lasagna noodles
1 8-ounce package frozen chopped spinach
½ cup low-sodium chicken broth
1 large onion, chopped
½ green bell pepper, chopped
½ red bell pepper, chopped
3 garlic cloves, minced
⅛ teaspoon oregano
⅛ teaspoon thyme
⅛ teaspoon rosemary
⅛ teaspoon crushed red pepper
1 16-ounce jar low-fat spaghetti sauce
1 large eggplant, peeled and cut into ¼-inch slices
15 ounces low-fat ricotta cheese
1½ cups diced nonfat mozzarella cheese
½ cup grated nonfat Parmesan cheese
1 head lettuce
2 large tomatoes
¼ cup balsamic vinegar
2 cups carrots, cooked
2 cups chopped asparagus, cooked

1. Preheat oven to 350°F.
2. Cook lasagna noodles according to package directions. Drain and set aside.
3. Cook spinach according to package directions.
4. In a large pot, "sauté" the onion, peppers, spinach, and garlic in chicken broth for 5 minutes, or until onion is slightly soft.
5. Add oregano, thyme, rosemary, and crushed red pepper. Mix well. Stir in sauce and mix well. Cover and simmer for 15 minutes.

6. In a large nonstick frying pan, fry eggplant until browned on both sides.

7. Distribute one-fourth of the sauce over the bottom of a 9 × 13-inch baking dish. Place one-third of the lasagna noodles over the sauce. Put half the eggplant over the noodles. Place half the ricotta and mozzarella over the eggplant.

8. Repeat layers, ending with the lasagna noodles and remaining sauce.

9. Top with Parmesan cheese sprinkled evenly over tomato sauce. Cover and bake for 40 minutes.

10. Prepare tossed salad, breaking up lettuce and cutting tomatoes into eighths. Sprinkle salad with balsamic vinegar.

11. Serve lasagne with salad, carrots, and asparagus.

Lasagne
Calories: 738
Protein: 77 g
Fat: 11 g
Sodium: 1756 mg
Cholesterol: 72 mg

Carrots and Asparagus
Calories: 47
Protein: 3.3 g
Fat: 0.9 g
Sodium: 25 mg
Cholesterol: 0

Tossed Salad
Calories: 43 g
Protein: 2.2 g
Fat: 0.5 g
Sodium: 9 mg
Cholesterol: 0

23. Confidence Chicken Cacciatore and Peas

Serves 4

1 32-ounce can whole Italian tomatoes
1 4-ounce can tomato paste
1 onion, halved, sliced, and separated
2 cups water
4 skinless whole chicken breasts, with bone
1 bay leaf
½ teaspoon oregano
⅛ teaspoon rosemary
¾ teaspoon garlic powder
¾ teaspoon onion powder
½ cup red wine
2⅔ cups cooked instant brown rice
4 cups peas, cooked

1. In a large pot, place the tomatoes, tomato paste, onion, and water. Mix thoroughly, crushing the tomatoes with a fork.
2. Add the chicken, seasonings, and wine and mix thoroughly.
3. Bring to a boil, reduce heat to medium-low, and cook for 25 to 30 minutes, or until chicken is cooked through.
4. Serve with rice and peas on the side.

Chicken
Calories: 497
Protein: 77 g
Fat: 10 g
Sodium: 204 mg
Cholesterol: 195

Brown Rice
Calories: 119
Protein: 2.5 g
Fat: 0.6 g
Sodium: 2 mg
Cholesterol: 0

Peas
Calories: 126
Protein: 10 g
Fat: 0.6 g
Sodium: 702 mg
Cholesterol: 0 mg

24. Hungry Woman's Halibut, Brown Rice, and Carrots

Serves 3

1 cup oat-bran cereal
¼ cup minced red bell pepper
¼ cup finely chopped onion
¼ cup finely chopped celery
1 egg white
2 tablespoons orange juice
3 6-ounce pieces of halibut fillet
2 cups cooked instant brown rice
3 cups sliced carrots, cooked

1. Preheat oven to 350°F.
2. Mix the cereal, red pepper, onion, and celery. Add the egg white and orange juice and combine thoroughly.
3. Pour the mixture onto a flat plate. Bread-coat the fish on both sides.
4. Bake for 20 minutes, or until fish flakes.
5. Serve with brown rice and carrots on the side.

Fish
Calories: 329
Protein: 42 g
Fat: 4.9 g
Sodium: 306 mg
Cholesterol: 91 mg

Brown Rice
Calories: 119
Protein: 2.5 g
Fat: 0.6 g
Sodium: 2 mg
Cholesterol: 0

Carrots
Calories: 47
Protein: 1.4 g
Fat: 0.2 g
Sodium: 50 mg
Cholesterol: 0

25. Squid-Squeeze Fettuccine with Mushrooms and Tomatoes

Serves 4

1 onion, thinly sliced
¼ cup low-sodium chicken broth
¼ cup white wine
1 teaspoon salt
⅛ teaspoon pepper
⅛ teaspoon paprika
½ cup 1% milk
½ teaspoon lime juice
8 ounces diced cooked squid (or shrimp)
3½ cups cooked fettuccine
¼ cup grated nonfat Parmesan cheese
2 cups sliced fresh mushrooms, sautéed
3 large tomatoes, sliced
1 teaspoon oregano
Sprinkle of wine vinegar

1. "Sauté" the onion in the chicken broth over high heat for 5 minutes, or until nearly soft.

2. Add wine, salt, pepper, paprika, and milk and bring to a boil. Lower heat and, stirring constantly, simmer for 25 minutes, uncovered.

3. Add lime juice and squid and combine thoroughly.

4. Gently stir in fettuccine, then sprinkle with Parmesan cheese.

5. Serve with mushrooms and tomatoes on the side, sprinkled with oregano and vinegar. (You can mix this in with the fettuccine instead.)

Fettuccine
Calories: 258
Protein: 18 g
Fat: 2.1 g
Sodium: 109 mg
Cholesterol: 152 mg

Mushrooms and Tomatoes
Calories: 54
Protein: 3.3 g
Fat: 0.7 g
Sodium: 7 mg
Cholesterol: 0

26. Barbara's Bull's-Eye Rice and Beans

Serves 6

4¼ cups water
2 packages Goya Sazón seasoning
2½ cups Vitarroz white rice (Spanish brand)
1 green bell pepper, chopped
2 red bell peppers, chopped
1 large onion, chopped
1 garlic clove, chopped
¼ cup chopped fresh parsley
¼ cup low-sodium chicken broth
¼ cup tomato sauce
1 16-ounce can Progresso kidney beans, rinsed and drained

1. Bring 4 cups of water to a boil, add Sazón seasoning and rice, and boil for 5 minutes. Lower heat to barely a simmer, cover, and cook for 15 minutes.

2. In a large nonstick frying pan, sauté the peppers, onion, garlic, and parsley in chicken broth for 5 minutes, or until onion is nearly soft.

3. Add tomato sauce and ¼ cup of water. Stir in the kidney beans.

4. Place rice in a large bowl and toss with kidney bean mixture. (Or, instead of draining and rinsing beans, place contents of can in a pot, add the ¼ cup water, tomato sauce, ⅛ teaspoon garlic powder, ⅛ teaspoon salt, and ⅛ teaspoon pepper. Heat thoroughly and serve in separate bowls to spoon on top of rice.)

Calories: 298
Protein: 10 g
Fat: 0.7
Sodium: 19 mg
Cholesterol: 0

27. Mother's Vegetable Delight with Sea Bass

Serves 6

5 onions, chopped
6 green bell peppers, chopped
2 red bell peppers, chopped
1 jalapeño pepper, seeded
2 teaspoons canola oil
2 cups tomato sauce
2 4-ounce cans sliced mushrooms
1 package Goya Sazón seasoning
1 package low-sodium beef broth mix
1 teaspoon garlic powder
1 teaspoon oregano
6 8-ounce sea bass fillets
Sprinkle of lemon juice
Sprinkle of pepper
Sprinkle of paprika
2 large heads green cabbage, cooked and shredded
3 cups sliced carrots, cooked

1. In a nonstick frying pan, sauté onions and peppers in the canola oil for 5 minutes, or until onions are nearly soft.

2. Add tomato sauce and mushrooms and mix thoroughly. Stir in Goya seasoning, beef broth mix, garlic powder, and oregano. Cook for 20 minutes. Let cool for 5 minutes.

3. Sprinkle the sea bass with lemon juice, pepper, and paprika and broil to taste (about 7 minutes).

4. Spoon ⅙ of the cabbage onto a plate and top with ⅙ of the onion-pepper-tomato-mushroom mix. Serve with carrots and sea bass.

Calories: 412
Protein: 58 g
Fat: 5.7 g
Sodium: 781 mg
Cholesterol: 140 mg

28. Orange-Pineapple Chicken with Brown Rice and Mushrooms

Serves 6

¼ cup orange juice
1 tablespoon low-sodium soy sauce
2 teaspoons dry sherry
1 teaspoon grated orange peel
1 tablespoon chopped canned pineapple, with ¼ cup juice
    reserved
1 small onion, thinly sliced
⅛ teaspoon garlic powder
⅛ teaspoon freshly ground pepper
1½ pounds boneless and skinless chicken breasts,
    cut into strips
24 large fresh mushrooms, sliced
2 cups green beans, cooked
2 tablespoons all-purpose flour
2⅔ cups cooked instant brown rice

1. Mix the orange juice, soy sauce, sherry, orange peel, chopped pineapple and reserved juice, onion, garlic powder, and pepper. Stir in chicken strips and mix thoroughly. Refrigerate for 30 minutes or overnight.

2. Broil the mushrooms for 6 minutes, until tender and juicy. Shut off broiler but leave mushrooms in to stay warm until ready for use.

3. Place a strainer over a bowl and pour chicken mixture into strainer. Save marinade.

4. In a large nonstick frying pan, cook chicken strips for 2 to 3 minutes, continually turning until slightly brown on all sides.

5. Stir in green beans and cook for 2 more minutes.

6. Mix flour into marinade and stir until thoroughly blended.

Immediately pour into frying pan and boil until sauce thickens, stirring constantly.

7. Serve with brown rice and broiled mushrooms.

Note: You can also mix the rice and/or mushrooms into the chicken combination.

Chicken
Calories: 354
Protein: 57 g
Fat: 6.2 g
Sodium: 236 mg
Cholesterol: 146 mg

Mushrooms
Calories: 60
Protein: 4.2 g
Fat: 0.8 g
Sodium: 8 mg
Cholesterol: 0

Brown Rice
Calories: 119
Protein: 2.5 g
Fat: 0.6 g
Sodium: 2 mg
Cholesterol: 0

29. Shrimp-Vegetable Peak Contraction Pasta
Serves 4

1 pound Jerusalem artichoke linguine or regular linguine
1 cup chopped green onions
1 red bell pepper, chopped
1 green bell pepper, chopped
4 fresh mushrooms, chopped
3 tomatoes, chopped
¼ cup low-sodium chicken broth
10 jumbo shrimp, chopped
¼ teaspoon garlic powder
¼ teaspoon oregano
¼ teaspoon thyme
⅛ teaspoon basil
⅛ teaspoon crushed pepper
1 teaspoon parsley
3 cups mixed vegetables (from frozen package)
2 tablespoons rice vinegar
½ cup grated nonfat Parmesan cheese

1. Cook linguine according to package directions. Drain and place in mixing bowl. Set aside.
2. In a nonstick skillet, sauté green onions, peppers, mushrooms, and tomatoes in chicken broth over high heat for 5 minutes, or until green onions are nearly soft.
3. Add shrimp and seasonings and mix thoroughly.
4. Stir in mixed vegetables and rice vinegar and stir thoroughly.
5. Spoon vegetable mixture over the linguine and sprinkle with Parmesan cheese.

Calories: 593
Protein: 29 g
Fat: 2.9 g
Sodium: 208 mg
Cholesterol: 37 mg

30. Spicy Mahimahi with Brown Rice and Cauliflower
Serves 2

1 tablespoon paprika
2 teaspoons oregano
2 teaspoons thyme
2 teaspoons garlic powder
1 teaspoon onion powder
⅛ teaspoon saffron
⅛ teaspoon fennel seeds
⅛ teaspoon rosemary
¼ teaspoon black pepper
⅛ teaspoon crushed red pepper
1½ pounds mahimahi fillets
2 teaspoons canola oil (optional)
2⅓ cups cooked brown rice
4 cups cauliflower florets, cooked

1. Preheat broiler.
2. Combine seasonings in a small bowl, then pour onto a large plate.
3. Brush the fish with oil on both sides. Press fish into spice mixture until completely coated on both sides.
4. Broil 4 to 5 inches from heat for 6 to 8 minutes, or until fish flakes when touched with a fork.
5. Add remaining seasoning mix to brown rice and serve with fish and cauliflower.

Note: The portion is very large—you may choose to cut it in half.

Fish
Calories: 425
Protein: 64 g
Fat: 3.2 g
Sodium: 301 mg
Cholesterol: 248 mg

Brown Rice
Calories: 119
Protein: 2.5 g
Fat: 0.6 g
Sodium: 2 mg
Cholesterol: 0

Cauliflower
Calories: 25
Protein: 2.6 g
Fat: 0.2 g
Sodium: 10 mg
Cholesterol: 0

Canola Oil
Calories: 38
Protein: 0
Fat: 4.2 g
Sodium: 0
Cholesterol: 0

31. Runner's Rice and Black Beans with Okra

Serves 2

1 onion, chopped
1 tomato, chopped
2 garlic cloves, chopped
¼ teaspoon dry mustard
½ teaspoon chili powder
½ teaspoon salt
2 whole cloves
1 bay leaf
2 cups plain tomato sauce
1 cup cooked black beans (or drained canned rinsed beans)
2⅔ cups cooked instant brown rice
2 cups chopped okra (from frozen package), cooked

1. In a nonstick frying pan, sauté onion, tomato, and garlic for 5 minutes, or until onion is nearly soft.

2. Mix in mustard, chili powder, salt, cloves, and bay leaf and cook for 1 minute.

3. Add tomato sauce and bring to a boil. Lower heat and add beans. Simmer for 1 minute.

4. Serve over a bed of brown rice with okra on the side, or mix beans into the rice.

Beans
Calories: 457
Protein: 19 g
Fat: 2.3 g
Sodium: 188 mg
Cholesterol: 0

Okra
Calories: 58
Protein: 4 g
Fat: 0.6 g
Sodium: 4 mg
Cholesterol: 0

CHAPTER EIGHT

SNACK MENUS FOR A MONTH

Snacking—it's the story of my life! Even now, as I write, I'm snacking. I'm a grazer at heart. If I'm home all day, and I'm in an eating mood, look out! I snack all day.

With the eating plan in this book, you are allowed to eat more than five times a day. But you are *required* to eat at least five times a day—three low-fat meals plus two low-fat snacks. The reason for this is explained in Chapter 3.

In the following pages, I offer sixty-two snacks—two a day for a month. The first thirty-one snacks are quickies. Where preparation is necessary, the work is obvious so I won't give directions. For example, I'm not going to tell you to "cut the bagel and spread the cream cheese." *These all serve 1.* The remaining snacks take a little longer to prepare, but not so long as to discourage you. Even lazy Joyce prepares them quite often!

UNDERSTANDING THE NUTRITIONAL INFORMATION

Following each recipe are one or more nutritional analyses listing the calorie content plus protein, fat, sodium, and carbohydrate found in the food. The calculations are *per serving* unless otherwise indicated. For example, in a recipe serving four persons, the analysis will be for one serving. For a recipe yielding twenty cookies, four cookies constituting a serving, the analysis will be for four cookies.

You will note that when an item is added as an accompaniment, the calculations are shown separately—one analysis for the main item and one for the accompaniment—so that you have detailed information on the food values of the specific foods you are eating. Also, if you are using the recipes to make up your own meal plans, you might want to eliminate or substitute the accompaniments.

Protein and fat measures are shown in grams (g); sodium and carbohydrate contents are given in milligrams (mg). Refer to Chapter 3 for guidelines on using these figures. Bear in mind, however, that the meal plans in Chapter 9 count everything for you—these analyses are for your information in case you want to make your own daily meal plans.

When an alternative ingredient appears in parentheses, this means the substitute has not been included in the analysis. For example, "1 teaspoon garlic powder (or salt)" means that the analysis includes garlic powder but not salt (which would yield a higher sodium content).

When recipes include wheat germ or canola oil, the analysis for these items is usually kept separate. I've added these items in the recipe to meet the fat requirements in the meal plans, but if you are developing your own meal plans, you might want to omit these items and obtain your fat minimum in another way. In the rare cases when it is included in the recipe, it is because I feel it is absolutely necessary to the taste of the recipe.

A NOTE ABOUT THE RECIPES

Where nonstick cookware is involved, it is assumed that you have lightly coated the cookware with a vegetable oil cooking spray, like Pam.

When 1 percent dairy products are used, feel free to substitute nonfat products. I use the 1 percent items when I feel you need that bit of fat to fulfill a healthy daily fat requirement. (The minimum fat you should get is 10 percent of total caloric intake.)

Fruits and vegetables in the ingredients lists are medium size unless otherwise indicated. Herbs and spices are dried unless fresh is indicated.

When I list a particular vegetable snack, feel free to change it to an equivalent vegetable snack. For example, if the snack is an unlimited complex carbohydrate vegetable, such as broccoli, you can exchange it for any other *unlimited* complex carbohydrate, such as cauliflower or green beans. If it is a limited vegetable, such as corn, you can exchange it for another *limited* vegetable, such as potatoes, yams, or beets. The same goes for any other snack, such as fruits or breads.

QUICKIE SNACKS

1. Bagel and Cream Cheese with Plums

½ plain bagel
1 tablespoon low-fat cream cheese
2 plums

Bagel
Calories: 102
Protein: 4.8 g
Fat: 1.4 g
Sodium: 242 mg
Cholesterol: 0

Cream Cheese
Calories: 30
Protein: 1.5 g
Fat: 2.5 g
Sodium: 80 mg
Cholesterol: 8 mg

Plums
Calories: 66
Protein: 0.5 g
Fat: 0
Sodium: 2 mg
Cholesterol: 0

2. Corn on the Cob with Butter Buds

1 ear corn
Butter Buds

Calories: 100
Protein: 3.3 g
Fat: 1 g
Sodium: 1 mg
Cholesterol: 0

3. Minestrone Soup

1 16-ounce can Pritikin Minestrone soup (or any other
low-fat soup)

Calories: 160
Protein: 8 g
Fat: 2 g
Sodium: 270 mg
Cholesterol: 0

4. Apple Jacks Candy

1 cup Kellogg's Apple Jacks (or any low-fat cereal)

Calories: 110
Protein: 2 g
Fat: 0.4 g
Sodium: 135 mg
Cholesterol: 0

5. Baked Potato with Mustard

1 large baking potato, baked and cooled
Mustard

Calories: 232
Protein: 6.9 g
Fat: 1.2 g
Sodium: 204 mg
Cholesterol: 0

6. Watermelon and Strawberries

1 wedge watermelon
1 cup strawberries

Calories: 222
Protein: 4.2 g
Fat: 2.8 g
Sodium: 13 mg
Cholesterol: 0

7. Peach Yogurt

1 6-ounce container nonfat peach yogurt

Calories: 90
Protein: 5 g
Fat: 0
Sodium: 85 mg
Cholesterol: 5 mg

Note: As an alternative, try 1% 8-ounce fruit yogurt (any flavor). Analysis is as follows:

Calories: 225
Protein: 9 g
Fat: 2.6 g
Sodium: 121 mg
Cholesterol: 10 mg

8. Raisins

1½ ounces raisins

Calories: 119
Protein: 1.3 g
Fat: 0.2 g
Sodium: 5 mg
Cholesterol: 0

9. Raw Vegetable Plate

1 each carrot, celery stalk, red bell pepper, tomato, and cucumber
Wine vinegar
Salt and pepper

Calories: 102
Protein: 3.9 g
Fat: 0.8 g
Sodium: 90 mg
Cholesterol: 0

10. Broccoli and Cauliflower

1½ cups each steamed cauliflower and broccoli

Calories: 116
Protein: 13 g
Fat: 1.2 g
Sodium: 45 mg
Cholesterol: 0

11. Cinnamon-Apple Oatmeal

1.25 ounces (½ cup dry) Quaker Cinnamon Apple Oatmeal

Calories: 120
Protein: 4 g
Fat: 2 g
Sodium: 100 mg
Cholesterol: 0

12. V-8 Juice

5.5-ounce can low-sodium V-8 juice

Calories: 53
Protein: 1.3 g
Fat: 0
Sodium: 67 mg
Cholesterol: 0

13. Egg White Sandwich

4 hard-boiled egg whites
½ onion, chopped
2 tablespoons nonfat mayonnaise
2 slices whole wheat toast
1 lettuce leaf

Calories: 228
Protein: 18 g
Fat: 1.5 g
Sodium: 435 mg
Cholesterol: 1 mg

14. Pretzels

2 large hard nonfat low-sodium pretzels or 15 thin ones

Calories: 110
Protein: 3 g
Fat: 0
Sodium: 350 mg
Cholesterol: 0

Note: Divide the package by its total servings and put the pretzels in plastic Baggies of one serving each.

15. Popcorn

½ envelope Orville Redenbacher's Smart Pop

Calories: 150
Protein: 4.5 g
Fat: 4.5 g
Sodium: 680 mg
Cholesterol: 0

Note: Pop the corn in microwave oven according to directions.

16. ½ Cup Frozen Yogurt

½ cup nonfat frozen yogurt

Calories: 151
Protein: 5 g
Fat: 0 g
Sodium: 83 mg
Cholesterol: 0

17. Peas and Carrots

2 cups peas and carrots (from frozen package)

Calories: 176
Protein: 11 g
Fat: 0.8 g
Sodium: 280 mg
Cholesterol: 0

18. English Muffin Pizza

½ whole-grain English muffin
¼ cup grated nonfat cheddar cheese
⅛ cup low-fat tomato sauce

Calories: 105
Protein: 11 g
Fat: 1.1 g
Sodium: 373 mg
Cholesterol: 5 mg

19. Rice Cakes

3 average plain rice cakes

Calories: 105
Protein: 2.1 g
Fat: 0.6
Sodium: 42 mg
Cholesterol: 0

20. Graham Crackers

2 large fat-free honey graham crackers or 1 serving
   SnackWell's Fat-Free Cinnamon Graham Snacks

Calories: 107
Protein: 1.7 g
Fat: 3 g
Sodium: 131 mg
Cholesterol: 0

21. Angel Food Cake or Cupcakes

1 slice angel food cake or 1 nonfat cupcake

Calories: 117
Protein: 2.6 g
Fat: 0
Sodium: 66 mg
Cholesterol: 0

22. Tomato and Lettuce Sandwich

1 tomato, sliced
1 lettuce leaf
2 slices Wonder Lite whole wheat bread, toasted
1 tablespoon nonfat mayonnaise

Calories: 111
Protein: 6.1 g
Fat: 1.5 g
Sodium: 344 mg
Cholesterol: 0

23. Baked Sweet Potato

1 large sweet potato, baked

Calories: 254
Protein: 3.8 g
Fat: 0.9 g
Sodium: 22 mg
Cholesterol: 0

24. Sliced Tomatoes on a Pita

1 tomato, sliced
1 whole wheat pita loaf
2 tablespoons nonfat salad dressing

Calories: 151
Protein: 5.5 g
Fat: 0.9 g
Sodium: 219 mg
Cholesterol: 0

25. Frozen Tangerines

3 tangerines, separated into sections and frozen

Calories: 66
Protein: 0.9 g
Fat: 0.3 g
Sodium: 2 mg
Cholesterol: 0

26. Broiled Pepper, Onion, Tomato, and Mushrooms

1 large red bell pepper, sliced
1 tomato, sliced
1 onion, sliced
5 mushrooms, sliced

Calories: 130
Protein: 6.6 g
Fat: 1.3 g
Sodium: 19 mg
Cholesterol: 0

Note: Season to taste and broil on aluminum foil for 6 minutes.

27. Rice and Chicken Broth

1 cup low-sodium chicken broth
½ cup uncooked instant white rice

Calories: 115
Protein: 3.2 g
Fat: 0.1 g
Sodium: 78 mg
Cholesterol: 0

Note: Boil water; add chicken broth and rice; let sit 2 minutes.

28. Jerusalem Artichokes

2 Jerusalem artichokes

Calories: 82
Protein: 4.6 g
Fat: 0.2 g
Sodium: 0
Cholesterol: 0

29. Raspberry Sorbet

⅓ cup raspberry sorbet

Calories: 60
Protein: 0
Fat: 0
Sodium: 37 mg
Cholesterol: 0

30. Lettuce and Tomato Salad

½ head lettuce
1 tomato, sliced
Wine vinegar

Calories: 47
Protein: 2.1 g
Fat: 0.5 g
Sodium: 11 mg
Cholesterol: 0

31. Pickle-Pepper Salad

¼ head lettuce
2 tablespoons chopped pickles
½ red bell pepper, diced

1. Break up lettuce and place in bowl.
2. Add pickles and pepper and combine thoroughly.

Calories: 30
Protein: 1 g
Fat: 0
Sodium: 176 mg
Cholesterol: 0

NOT-QUITE-SO-QUICK SNACKS

32. Baked Athletic Cinnamon-Raisin Squash with Cottage Cheese

Serves 2

1 medium to large acorn squash
1 tablespoon water
⅛ teaspoon cinnamon
Sprinkle of nutmeg
Sprinkle of artificial sweetener (optional)
½ cup seedless raisins
1 cup 1% cottage cheese

    1. Preheat oven to 350°F.
    2. Cut squash in half and remove seeds. Pierce squash on inside 10 times, add ½ tablespoon of water to each half, and sprinkle each with cinnamon, nutmeg, and sweetener.
    3. Fill each squash half with half the raisins.
    4. Wrap in aluminum foil and bake for 30 minutes, or until tender. (Or wrap in microwave-safe plastic wrap and bake for 5 minutes on high in microwave.)
    4. Serve with ½ cup cottage cheese on the side.

Squash
Calories: 206
Protein: 2.9 g
Fat: 0
Sodium: 11 mg
Cholesterol: 0

Cottage Cheese
Calories: 82
Protein: 14 g
Fat: 1.2 g
Sodium: 461 mg
Cholesterol: 6 mg

33. Punchy Parsnips

Serves 2

2 parsnips
½ cup Italian bread crumbs

1. Peel parsnips and cut into slices.
2. Steam 10 minutes in steamer, or until tender. (Or cover in plastic wrap and cook in microwave on high for 3 minutes.) Preheat oven to 350°F.
3. Puree in food processor and place in small ovenproof dish.
4. Sprinkle with bread crumbs and bake until lightly browned, about 20 minutes, or microwave on high for 3 minutes.

Calories: 167
Protein: 5.2 g
Fat: 1.6 g
Sodium: 150 mg
Cholesterol: 1 mg

Note: Add an optional 1 tablespoon grated nonfat cheddar cheese before baking.

34. Rousing Rutabaga

Serves 1

2 rutabagas (yellow turnips)
½ cup low-sodium chicken broth
½ teaspoon chopped fresh parsley

1. Peel and cut rutabagas into ½-inch-thick slices.

2. In a nonstick pan, cook rutabagas in broth until tender, appoximately 20 minutes. Don't overcook.

3. Sprinkle with parsley and serve hot.

Calories: 147
Protein: 4.8 g
Fat: 0
Sodium: 95 mg
Cholesterol: 0

35. Sweet Cinnamon-Apple Toast

Serves 1

1 apple, cored, unpeeled, and thinly sliced
¼ cup applesauce
⅛ teaspoon cinnamon
⅛ teaspoon nutmeg
⅛ teaspoon brown sugar
2 slices whole wheat bread, toasted

1. Preheat oven to 450°F.

2. In a nonstick frying pan, combine apple, applesauce, cinnamon, nutmeg, and brown sugar. Mix thoroughly. Cook for 5 minutes, stirring continually.

3. Spread mixture over toast. Bake for 3 minutes, then serve hot.

Calories: 230
Protein: 5.2 g
Fat: 2.2 g
Sodium: 246 mg
Cholesterol: 1 mg

36. Peach–Cottage Cheese Pick-Me-Up

Serves 1

1 peach
1 cup nonfat unsalted cottage cheese

1. Cut peach in half lengthwise and remove pit. Remove insides from peach halves, creating cavities for the cottage cheese.
2. Fill cavities with cottage cheese to overflowing.

Note: You may eat the leftover cottage cheese if it does not fill the peach halves.

Calories: 223
Protein: 33 g
Fat: 0.1 g
Sodium: 101 mg
Cholesterol: 20 mg

37. Lucky Vanilla-Lemon Lift Cookies and Milk

Makes 20 cookies, 4 cookies per serving

1 cup all-purpose flour
2 teaspoons baking soda
¼ cup applesauce
6 packets artificial sweetener
½ teaspoon grated lemon peel
⅛ teaspoon vanilla extract
3 egg whites
8-ounce glass 1% milk (see Note)

1. Preheat oven to 350°F.

2. Mix the flour and baking soda and set aside.

3. In a large mixer bowl, combine applesauce, artificial sweetener, lemon peel, and vanilla extract. Beat on medium speed until fully combined.

4. Add in egg whites and beat until fully blended.

5. Slowly add flour mixture, beating until well blended.

6. On a nonstick cookie sheet, drop generous teaspoonfuls to form the cookies, spacing about 2 inches apart.

7. Bake for 7 minutes, or until cookies are lightly browned.

8. Let cool and serve, or serve piping hot, with a glass of milk on the side.

Note: You can eliminate the milk or substitute nonfat milk.

Cookies (4)
Calories: 150
Protein: 6.1 g
Fat: 0.4 g
Sodium: 446 mg
Cholesterol: 0

Milk
Calories: 102
Protein: 8 g
Fat: 2.6 g
Sodium: 123 mg
Cholesterol: 10 mg

38. Before and After Blueberry Pineapple Pita Treat

Serves 1

¼ cup diced pineapple
1 cup blueberries
¼ cup applesauce
¼ teaspoon cinnamon
¼ teaspoon nutmeg
2 packets artificial sweetener
⅛ teaspoon vanilla extract
1 whole wheat pita bread

1. In a large nonstick skillet, combine pineapple, blueberries, applesauce, cinnamon, nutmeg, sweetener, and vanilla. Cook over medium heat, stirring constantly, for 4 minutes.

2. Pour into pita bread. Heat in microwave for 1 minute on high.

3. Wait 3 minutes, then serve piping hot or serve cold.

Note: This fruit mix is good over fat-free ice cream.

Calories: 258
Protein: 5.7 g
Fat: 1.8 g
Sodium: 227 mg
Cholesterol: 0

39. Island Treat Strawberry Ice Cream

Serves 2

2 cups halved strawberries
2 tablespoons nonfat dry milk
6 ice cubes
¼ teaspoon vanilla extract
¼ teaspoon almond extract
4 packages artificial sweetener

1. Place strawberries in a food processor and blend until smooth.

2. Add nonfat dry milk and mix thoroughly.

3. Stir in ice cubes, extracts, and sweetener and blend until smooth. Serve immediately.

Calories: 60
Protein: 1.6 g
Fat: 0.6 g
Sodium: 9 mg
Cholesterol: 0

40. Crunchy Cherry-Strawberry Yogurt Treat

Serves 1

4 ounces low-fat strawberry yogurt
½ cup chopped cherries
½ cup cornflakes

1. Place a layer of yogurt in the bottom of a dessert dish.

2. Put a layer of chopped cherries on top of the yogurt.

3. Place a layer of cornflakes on top of the cherries.

4. Repeat until you use up the mixture. Serve immediately or refrigerate 1 hour and then serve.

Calories: 244
Protein: 6.7 g
Fat: 2.8 g
Sodium: 70 mg
Cholesterol: 5 mg

41. Baked Raisin-Apple-Rum Delight

Serves 4

½ cup bran cereal, crushed
4 packets artificial sweetener
¼ cup all-purpose flour
2 teaspoons baking powder
⅛ teaspoon cinnamon
⅛ teaspoon nutmeg
1 cup diced apple
2 egg whites
¼ teaspoon rum extract
¼ teaspoon vanilla extract
¼ cup raisins

1. Preheat oven to 325°F.
2. Combine bran cereal, sweetener, flour, baking powder, cinnamon, and nutmeg. Mix thoroughly and stir in apple.
3. Add egg whites and extracts and mix thoroughly.
4. Pour mixture into 9-inch nonstick pie plate and sprinkle with raisins.
5. Bake for 25 minutes, or until lightly browned. Serve warm or cold.

Calories: 119
Protein: 3.8 g
Fat: 0.6 g
Sodium: 249 mg
Cholesterol: 0

42. Luscious Lentil Salad

Serves 2

½ head lettuce
1 large tomato, cut into eighths
1 radish, chopped
½ onion, thinly sliced
½ cup cooked lentils
2 fresh mushrooms, sliced
½ lemon
Dash of pepper
Dash of salt
1 tablespoon chopped fresh cilantro
1 tablespoon chopped fresh mint

1. Break up lettuce into a large bowl.
2. Add tomato, radish, onion, lentils, and mushrooms. Toss well.
3. Squeeze lemon juice into salad and toss again.
4. Add pepper, salt, cilantro, and mint. Toss and serve.

Calories: 149
Protein: 9.2 g
Fat: 0.7 g
Sodium: 82 mg
Cholesterol: 0

43. Joyce's Peppy Potato Salad

Serves 2

4 small red potatoes, cooked
2 onions, chopped
1 shallot, minced
1 celery stalk, minced
½ garlic clove, minced
½ teaspoon dill
½ teaspoon chives
⅔ cup nonfat plain yogurt mixed with 2 tablespoons lemon
    juice
Sprinkle of pepper
Sprinkle of paprika
Sprinkle of salt

1. Peel the potatoes and cut into cubes. Place in bowl.
2. Add onions, shallot, celery, garlic, dill, and chives and toss thoroughly.
3. Add yogurt–lemon juice mixture and toss thoroughly.
4. Sprinkle with pepper, paprika, and salt. Refrigerate 1 hour or more, then serve.

Calories: 329
Protein: 12 g
Fat: 0.5 g
Sodium: 155 mg
Cholesterol: 1.7 mg

44. Red-Eye Mashed Potatoes

Serves 2

1 large tomato, chopped
1 garlic clove, minced
¼ cup low-sodium chicken broth

½ cup nonfat buttermilk
½ cup skim milk
4 cooked peeled red potatoes
½ teaspoon dill
½ teaspoon parsley
Sprinkle of oregano
Sprinkle of paprika
Sprinkle of pepper
¼ teaspoon salt

1. In a small nonstick frying pan, "sauté" tomato and garlic in the chicken broth over high heat for 5 minutes. Set aside.

2. Mix the buttermilk and skim milk in a saucepan. Over low heat, warm the milk but don't let boil.

3. Place potatoes in a large bowl and add tomato mixture. Toss.

4. Sprinkle with seasonings and toss. Stir in milk and toss. Serve hot.

Calories: 265
Protein: 9 g
Fat: 0.7 g
Sodium: 157 mg
Cholesterol: 2 mg

45. Sinful Sweet Potato Slices

Serves 4

4 sweet potatoes, sliced
Generous sprinkling of cinnamon and nutmeg
2 packets artificial sweetener

1. Preheat oven to 400°F.

2. Spread potato slices over a nonstick cookie sheet.

3. Sprinkle with a few drops of water, then with cinnamon, nutmeg, and sweetner.

4. Bake for 30 minutes, or until slices turn slightly crisp. Serve hot.

Calories: 262
Protein: 4 g
Fat: 0.9 g
Sodium: 22 mg
Cholesterol: 0

46. Energizing Eggplant-Tomato-Mushroom Bake

Serves 2

1 eggplant, sliced
1 teaspoon olive oil
2 large tomatoes, sliced
8 fresh mushrooms, sliced
½ cup low-fat tomato sauce
½ cup Italian-flavored bread crumbs

1. Preheat oven to 350°F.
2. On a large nonstick cookie sheet, arrange eggplant slices. Brush a drop or two of oil on each piece and rub in. Place a slice of tomato on top of each eggplant slice and one or two slices of mushroom on top of the tomato.
3. Spoon a few drops of sauce over each, then sprinkle with bread crumbs.
4. Bake for 25 minutes, then serve hot.

Calories: 214
Protein: 10 g
Fat: 4.4 g
Sodium: 161 mg
Cholesterol: 1 mg

47. Succulent Sautéed Soy Vegetables and Swordfish

Serves 2

1 tomato, sliced
4 fresh mushrooms, sliced
1 onion, sliced
1 yellow summer squash, sliced
1 zucchini, sliced
½ cup broccoli florets
¼ cup grated carrots
⅓ cup low-sodium soy sauce
2 tablespoons garlic-flavored red wine vinegar
¼ cup water, as needed
8 ounces swordfish steak, cooked and cut into chunks

1. In a large nonstick frying pan, "sauté" the vegetables in soy sauce and vinegar over high heat until nearly soft, adding water if necessary.

2. Add swordfish, stir, and transfer mixture to a bowl.

3. Serve immediately or refrigerate and serve cold.

Vegetables
Calories: 131
Protein: 8.8 g
Fat: 0.9 g
Sodium: 1958 mg
Cholesterol: 0

Swordfish
Calories: 197
Protein: 32 g
Fat: 6.9 g
Sodium: 152 mg
Cholesterol: 91 mg

Note: You can also make this recipe without the swordfish, which is why the fish analysis is separate.

48. Winter Squash and Broccoli Steambath

Serves 2

1 winter squash, such as acorn, peeled and cubed
1 cup chopped broccoli florets
¼ cup apple juice concentrate
1 tablespoon cornstarch
⅛ teaspoon dill

1. Steam squash and broccoli for 15 minutes.
2. In a small saucepan, mix apple juice concentrate, cornstarch, and dill. Cook over low heat until it thickens, stirring constantly.
3. Spread sauce over squash-broccoli combination. Serve hot.

Calories: 269
Protein: 8.7 g
Fat: 1.5 g
Sodium: 15 mg
Cholesterol: 0

49. Italian Vegetable Salad

Serves 2

½ head lettuce
6 small plum tomatoes, sliced
2 small green onions, thinly sliced
½ cup Italian green beans (from frozen package)
¼ cup nonfat cottage cheese
2 tablespoons skim milk
¼ cup nonfat yogurt
¼ teaspoon garlic powder
⅛ teaspoon oregano
⅛ teaspoon rosemary
Sprinkle of pepper

1. Break up lettuce into a large bowl.

2. Add tomatoes, green onions, and beans and toss.

3. In a separate bowl, combine cottage cheese, skim milk, and yogurt. Mix thoroughly and add spices. Mix again.

4. Pour mixture onto lettuce and toss thoroughly.

Calories: 104
Protein: 10 g
Fat: 0.7 g
Sodium: 45 mg
Cholesterol: 3 mg

50. Self-Confidence Caesar Salad

Serves 2

½ head romaine lettuce
2 tomatoes, cut into eighths
1 onion, thinly sliced
6 fresh mushrooms, sliced
⅛ teaspoon parsley
⅛ teaspoon black pepper
2 tablespoons wine vinegar
3 egg whites or ¼ cup Egg Beaters
1 tablespoon Dijon mustard
½ teaspoon garlic powder
1 tablespoon lime juice
1 tablespoon grated nonfat Parmesan cheese

1. In a large bowl, break up lettuce.

2. Add tomatoes, onion, mushrooms, parsley, and pepper.

3. In a separate bowl, mix vinegar, egg whites or Egg Beaters, mustard, garlic powder, lime juice, and cheese. Beat for 15 seconds.

4. Pour dressing over salad and toss thoroughly. Serve.

Note: If you add 4 to 6 ounces of diced cooked chicken or turkey breast, you have a whole meal here. Also note that since the egg whites would be raw, you may prefer Egg Beaters to avoid the possibility of salmonella poisoning.

Calories: 132
Protein: 11 g
Fat: 1.4 g
Sodium: 206 mg
Cholesterol: 3 mg

51. Cut-Up Carrot-Spinach Soup

Serves 4

1 red bell pepper, chopped
1 small onion, chopped
1 carrot, grated
1 tomato, diced
1 cup low-sodium beef broth
⅛ teaspoon garlic powder
2 cups low-sodium V-8 juice
8 ounces frozen chopped spinach, thawed
⅛ teaspoon lime juice
⅛ teaspoon crushed red pepper
1 tablespoon low-sodium soy sauce

1. In a nonstick frying pan, "sauté" red pepper, onion, carrot, and tomato in the beef broth over high heat until onion is soft.
2. Add garlic powder and mix thoroughly. Stir in V-8 juice and spinach and simmer for 8 minutes.
3. Add lime juice, red pepper, and soy sauce. Simmer for 4 minutes, then serve piping hot.

Calories: 64
Protein: 4.6 g
Fat: 0
Sodium: 212 mg
Cholesterol: 0

52. Tangy Romaine-Mushroom-Mustard Salad with a Pear

Serves 2

½ head romaine lettuce
7 fresh mushrooms, sliced
1 red onion, thinly sliced
1 tomato, diced
1 cucumber, diced
¼ cup red wine vinegar
2 tablespoons apple juice concentrate
¼ cup mustard
⅛ teaspoon paprika
⅛ teaspoon oregano
⅛ teaspoon garlic powder
⅛ teaspoon ginger
2 pears

1. Break up romaine lettuce into a large bowl. Add mushrooms, onion, tomato, and cucumber.
2. In a separate bowl, mix vinegar and apple juice concentrate. Add mustard and combine thoroughly. Stir in paprika, oregano, garlic powder, and ginger and mix well.
3. Pour dressing over salad and serve with pear on the side.

Salad
Calories: 132
Protein: 6.5 g
Fat: 2.4 g
Sodium: 393 mg
Cholesterol: 0

Pear
Calories: 118
Protein: 0.8 g
Fat: 0.8 g
Sodium: 0
Cholesterol: 0

53. Strut-Your-Stuff Green Bean Patties

Serves 4

10 egg whites
2 cups chopped French-cut green beans (thawed from frozen)
1½ cups Italian-flavored bread crumbs
¼ cup nonfat grated Parmesan cheese
⅛ teaspoon salt
⅛ teaspoon paprika
⅛ teaspoon garlic powder
⅛ teaspoon pepper

    1. In a large bowl, beat egg whites for about 30 seconds.
    2. In a large mixing bowl, combine beans, egg whites, bread crumbs, cheese, and seasonings. Mix thoroughly.
    3. Shape into 12 small patties.
    4. Cook patties in large nonstick skillet over medium heat for 1 to 2 minutes on each side. Serve hot.

Note: You may want to put some salsa on these patties.

Patties (3)
Calories: 171
Protein: 15 g
Fat: 1.3 g
Sodium: 406 mg
Cholesterol: 7 mg

54. Time-Out Tomato-Mushroom Snack

Serves 2

10 large fresh mushrooms, stems and caps separated
¼ cup chopped onion
½ cup chopped red bell pepper
1 cup chopped tomatoes

⅛ teaspoon garlic powder
⅛ teaspoon dill
3 tablespoons plain nonfat yogurt

1. Preheat oven to 350°F.
2. Chop the mushroom stems and set caps aside.
3. In a large nonstick frying pan, sauté onion, red pepper, and mushroom stems until the onion is nearly soft.
4. Add tomatoes, garlic powder, and dill and mix thoroughly. Cook for 1 more minute.
5. Remove pan from heat and blend in yogurt. Place the mushroom caps upside down. Fill each cap with the tomato mixture.
6. Bake for 8 minutes, then serve hot.

Calories: 97
Protein: 6.3 g
Fat: 1 g
Sodium: 28 mg
Cholesterol: 0.5 mg

55. Preconditioning Cherry-Rice Bake

Serves 4

1 egg white
2 cups cooked instant brown rice, cooled
½ teaspoon cinnamon
½ teaspoon nutmeg
4 ounces nonfat cream cheese
¼ cup nonfat sour cream
½ teaspoon rum extract
½ teaspoon vanilla extract
2 packets artificial sweetener
¼ cup applesauce
10 cherries, pitted and chopped

1. Preheat oven to 350°F.
2. Beat egg white lightly and set aside.
3. In a large bowl, mix rice, egg white, cinnamon, and nutmeg.
4. Pour into 8-inch nonstick baking pan and bake for 8 minutes.
5. In a separate bowl or food processor, combine cream cheese, sour cream, extracts, artificial sweetener, applesauce, and cherries.
6. Remove rice from oven and spread with topping. Cut into squares and serve.

Squares (2)
Calories: 155
Protein: 7.2 g
Fat: 0.8 g
Sodium: 184 mg
Cholesterol: 5 mg

56. Marvelous Melon-Strawberry Salad

Serves 4

1 head lettuce
½ cantaloupe, diced
¼ honeydew melon, diced
1 cup pineapple chunks
15 large strawberries, sliced
2 cups chopped cucumber

1. Break up lettuce into a large bowl.
2. Mix fruits and cucumber, toss with lettuce, and serve.

Calories: 97
Protein: 2.1 g
Fat: 0.6 g
Sodium: 18 mg
Cholesterol: 0

57. Bodybuilding Blueberry-Rum Rice Pudding

Serves 4

2 cups cooked white rice
2 packets artificial sweetener
1 cup 1% milk
1 cup vanilla nonfat yogurt
½ teaspoon vanilla extract
½ teaspoon rum extract
1 cup blueberries
Sprinkle of cinnamon

1. In a large pot, mix rice, sweetener, and milk. Stir thoroughly. Cook over medium heat for 10 minutes, stirring constantly.
2. Remove rice from heat and add yogurt, extracts, and blueberries.
3. Sprinkle with cinnamon. Serve hot or cold.

Calories: 192
Protein: 6.1 g
Fat: 1.5 g
Sodium: 63 mg
Cholesterol: 5 mg

58. Apple-Pear-Peach Salad

Serves 4

2 pears, cored and sliced
2 apples, cored and sliced
1 peach, pitted and sliced
4 teaspoons sesame seeds (optional)
Sprinkle of sugar (or artificial sweetener)

1. Place fruits and seeds in a large bowl and toss.
2. Sprinkle with sugar or sweetener and serve.

Calories: 115
Protein: 0.8 g
Fat: 0.7 g
Sodium: 1 mg
Cholesterol: 0

Sesame Seeds
Calories: 24
Protein: 1.1 g
Fat: 2.3 g
Sodium: 2 mg
Cholesterol: 0

59. Cranberry-Cherry Cottage Cheese Pudding

Serves 2

1 cup 1% cottage cheese
¼ cup nonfat sour cream
¼ cup cranberry juice
4 cherries

1. In a large mixing bowl, combine cottage cheese, sour cream, and juice. Stir until thoroughly blended.
2. Pour into dessert dishes and top with cherries.

Note: You can puree the ingredients in a food processor or blender for a smoother consistency. I like it with the rougher consistency.

Calories: 138
Protein: 16 g
Fat: 1.4 g
Sodium: 502 mg
Cholesterol: 6 mg

60. Raspberry-Peach Milkshake

Serves 4

1 cup 1% milk
¼ cup nonfat dry milk
2 packets artificial sweetener
1 cup raspberries
1 cup diced fresh peach
⅛ teaspoon vanilla extract
1 cup ice cubes

1. Place all ingredients in a food processor or blender and puree until very smooth.
2. Serve quickly or it will thin out.

Calories: 88
Protein: 4.5 g
Fat: 1.3 g
Sodium: 55 mg
Cholesterol: 3 mg

61. Mango-Strawberry Delight

Serves 4

1 large mango, cubed
10 large strawberries, chopped
1 cup orange juice
1 cup unsweetened pineapple juice
1 cup cranberry juice
1 cup sparkling water
1 cup ice cubes

1. Place all ingredients in a food processor or blender and puree until smooth.
2. Serve immediately or mixture will thin out.

Calories: 139
Protein: 1 g
Fat: 0.5 g
Sodium: 6 mg
Cholesterol: 0

62. Baked Apples

Serves 4

1 tablespoon apple juice concentrate
1 tablespoon orange juice concentrate
4 McIntosh apples, cored (not peeled)
⅛ teaspoon cinnamon
¼ cup raisins

1. Mix apple juice and orange juice concentrate and set aside.

2. Sprinkle apples with cinnamon.

3. Divide juice concentrate among the 4 apples, spooning an equal amount into each apple cavity. Add raisins to each cavity.

4. Place apples in a microwave dish large enough to accommodate the apples so that they don't touch each other. Cover with plastic wrap. Puncture wrap in 5 places.

5. Bake on high for 5 minutes. Wait 5 minutes before eating. Serve hot or cold.

Calories: 191
Protein: 1 g
Fat: 1.1 g
Sodium: 4 mg
Cholesterol: 0

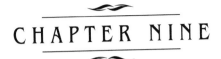

CHAPTER NINE

MEAL PLANS FOR A MONTH, DINING OUT, AND WORKING AROUND THE FAMILY

Okay. Here's what you've been requesting of me for years: a whole month's worth of meal plans that will allow you to eat plenty and lose weight without getting bored and while maintaining optimum nutrition. In the following pages, I've combined the breakfast, lunch, dinner, and snack menus into a month's worth of balanced eating.

You will note that the protein seems rather high at times. Well, it isn't if you consider that nearly every food item has some protein—even an orange or a cantaloupe. In other words, most of the time the high protein is the result of counting all the vegetable sources. Nutrition experts agree that high protein from these sources cannot harm you in any way; in fact, those who work out with weights crave higher-protein diets than those who do not. In menus that have a high protein count from animal sources, you decide whether you want to cut the protein portion in half or substitute beans or tofu. I must tell you that I—and the before-and-after people in this book—eat all the protein in these meal plans and thrive on it!

Note also that some of the meals fall short of the recommended 20 to 25 grams of fat. This is perfectly fine. The bare minimum of fat you should get is 12 to 18 grams—or 10 percent of your total calorie intake. To meet this requirement, sometimes I ask you to eat a 1 percent dairy product or add granola, sesame seeds, wheat germ, or canola oil. However, feel free to use the nonfat products and eliminate these items.

You will also note that, as a general rule, the total daily sodium measure is well below the USDA'S allowance of 2,500 to 3,000 milligrams. When this is the case, you may opt to add 1/4 teaspoon of salt, which amounts to 500 milligrams of sodium.

Cholesterol levels in these recipes are almost always well under the recommended 300 milligrams per day. When not, you can opt to eliminate the cholesterol culprit—here, it is the rare egg yolk I use.

Realize that I encourage you to eat even more vegetables than included in the meal plans. In other words, indulge as often as you please in the *unlimited complex carbohydrate* vegetables any time of any day. You need not calculate them into the plan, even though I have done so. (I did it so you would know the exact nutritional value of what you are eating on a daily basis.) Also, feel free to change the fruits or vegetables I offer in these plans.

In the following meal plans, men get to eat more because they are naturally more muscular due to the male's increased production of the hormone testosterone. The added muscle mass causes the metabolism to be higher and to burn more fat than a less muscular (female) person. If women work out with weights, they too can raise their metabolism, and eventually eat more without getting fat, but not as much as men.

There's no need to use all the recipes. You can double up on the ones you like or add some of your own. Finally, be creative! Start by using this month's meal plans, but then make your own using the guidelines in Chapter 3.

One more thing: Some of you will want to create meal plans

based solely on the quick and easy meals. You can do this by using the first ten recipes in each recipe chapter and the first thirty-one of the snack recipes.

MAKING YOUR OWN MEAL PLANS

In Chapter 3, I discussed how much fat, protein, simple unprocessed complex carbohydrate (fruit), limited complex carbohydrate (starches, grains), unlimited complex carbohydrate, and dairy you should eat for a healthy weight-loss eating plan. If you follow the meal plans here, you do not have to do any figuring; the calculations have all been done for you. Your daily requirements are fulfilled in the meal plans.

However, making your own plans is easy, too. You can go back to the breakfast, lunch, dinner, and snack chapters and make up your own daily meal plans. Just follow the guidelines in Chapter 3 (summarized below for your convenience) to make up your daily meal plans. Remember: You don't have to have every single component to the letter every day. In general, try to average them out over the week.

Also, for those who don't want to think about it, just take any breakfast, lunch, dinner, and two snacks to make up a meal plan. Without even thinking about the components, chances are your meal plan would be quite well balanced because you would automatically not choose, say, three fruity meals and two fruity snacks. Your own taste buds and common sense will guide you.

Nutritional Needs in a Nutshell

FAT   Women: 20–25 grams
                             Men: 30–40 grams

PROTEIN   Minimum 45 grams for women,
                             55 for men (see Chapter 3 for
                             serving sizes that compute grams)

SIMPLE UNPROCESSED   2–4 fruit (see Chapter 3 for list
CARBOHYDRATES   and serving sizes)

LIMITED COMPLEX   Women: 5–7 servings
CARBOHYDRATES   Men: 8–10 (Bread, grains,
                             cereal, rice, pasta, corn, beans,
                             peas, beets, lentils, potatoes;
                             see Chapter 3 for list and
                             serving sizes)

***UNLIMITED* COMPLEX**   6 or more 1/2-cup servings (all
CARBOHYDRATES   vegetables not in limited
                             category; see Chapter 3 for
                             list and serving sizes)

DAIRY   2–3 servings (see Chapter 3 for
                             list and serving sizes)

Note: For all foods, you can have less than the minimum on
any given day, but try not to go below *half* the minimum.

THE MEAL PLANS

Seven Important Reminders About the Meal Plans

1. The average daily caloric intake when calculated for the entire month is about 1500 and the fat grams are 18. All fat that reads "optional" has been included in the daily meal plans. That is, when you look up a given recipe in a meal plan, you may note that the canola oil, sesame seeds, wheat germ, and so forth is listed as optional. Your daily meal plan calculations *include* these items. I put it in to fulfill your daily fat requirements. If you leave them out you may *deduct* the calculations from your daily totals. The option comes when you are making your own daily meal plans—and mixing and matching the recipes.

2. Many of the portions are very large. If you feel you are eating too much, feel free to cut them by one-fourth, one-third, or even in half. But save the "cut" on the side. You may want it later (I'd rather you do that than be hungry and be tempted to cheat).

3. Try not to go below 10 percent of your daily caloric intake in fat. If you do, you will probably feel hungry all day, and have the constant urge to eat.

4. If you don't like animal protein, simply substitute that food in the meal plan with a bean or tofu meal.

5. The sodium content of the meals is very low. As noted on page 72, you may add salt to taste. One-quarter teaspoon of salt equals 500 milligrams of sodium.

6. Feel free to substitute any meal for any other meal in a daily meal plan scheme. Try to make it a comparable meal. You have all the calculations in the breakfast, lunch, dinner, and snack chapters.

7. I'm not concerned with the calories for the unlimited complex carbohydrates, even though they have been calculated into your daily meal plans and recipes. It's the *limited sim-*

ple and complex carbohydrates and the fat that you must watch. In other words, after you have eaten all of the food in your meal plan for the day, you can still have lettuce, carrots, celery, etc. Don't get bogged down with thinking, "This will add X amount of calories to my day." I calculated calories and other food values so you would know what you are eating, but I don't want you to think in terms of calories. Your fat is low and if you follow these meal plans, your calories are low enough to lose weight even if you go wild with the unlimited complex carbohydrates.

MEAL PLAN 1

Breakfast Joyce's Russian-French Toast (page 133)
Lunch   Weight-Training Turkey Burgers and Mozzarella Cheese on a Bun with Brussels Sprouts and Tossed Salad (page 173)
Dinner   Racy Fried Rice and Chicken with Zucchini (page 220)
Snacks   Before and After Blueberry Pineapple Pita Treat (page 262)
                Marvelous Melon-Strawberry Salad (page 276)

TOTALS FOR THE DAY
Calories: 1372
Protein: 96 g
Fat: 19 g
Sodium: 1372 mg
Cholesterol: 347 mg

MEAL PLAN 2

Breakfast Giant-Set Tomato-Cucumber Crepes with Orange Wedges (page 129) · 3 per serving
Lunch   Wonder Woman's White Wine Pasta with Salad (page 167) 1 g. per serving

Dinner   Poppy Joe's Sole Paella (page 217) 11 g.
Snacks   Baked Apples (page 280) 1.1 g.
           Punchy Parsnips (page 258) 1.6 g.

TOTALS FOR THE DAY
Calories: 1358
Protein: 62 g
Fat: 20 g
Sodium: 890 mg
Cholesterol: 102 mg

MEAL PLAN 3

Breakfast   1 Cup of Raisin Bran Cereal (page 126)
           1 cup raspberries
Lunch   Jump-Start Soup and Such (page 159)
Dinner   Broiled Chicken Breast with Carrots and White
           Rice (page 210)
Snacks   English Muffin Pizza (page 252)
           Frozen Tangerines (page 254)

TOTALS FOR THE DAY
Calories: 1261
Protein: 92 g
Fat: 17 g
Sodium: 1714 mg
Cholesterol: 191 mg

MEAL PLAN 4

Breakfast   Pita Pockets Power Omelet (page 132)
Lunch   Feather Kick-Up Fish Stew (page 172)
Dinner   Martha's Russian Cheese Blintzes and Broccoli
           (page 215)

Snacks   Sweet Cinnamon-Apple Toast (page 259)
              Island Treat Strawberry Ice Cream (page 262)
              Glass of 1% milk

TOTALS FOR THE DAY
Calories: 1404
Protein: 112 g
Fat: 22 g
Sodium: 2130 mg
Cholesterol: 259 mg

MEAL PLAN 5

Breakfast Nutty Nutmeg French Toast (page 134)
Lunch   Happy Muscle's Italian Chicken and Rice with
               Salad and Wheat Germ (page 170)
Dinner   Sporty Stuffed Red Peppers with Brussels Sprouts
               (page 219)
Snacks   Peach–Cottage Cheese Pick-Me-Up (page 260)
               Baked Raisin-Apple-Rum Delight (page 264)

TOTALS FOR THE DAY
Calories: 1601
Protein: 163 g
Fat: 18 g
Sodium: 1069 mg
Cholesterol: 224 mg

MEAL PLAN 6

Breakfast Poached Egg Push-Up with Raspberries (page 123)
Lunch   Mmm Mmm Good Microwave Baked Potatoes and
               Cottage Cheese with Green Beans (page 162)
Dinner   Broiled Sole and the Works with Capri Vegetables
               (page 208)

Snacks   Tomato and Lettuce Sandwich (page 253)
               Rice and Chicken Broth (page 255)
               1 cup broccoli

TOTALS FOR THE DAY
Calories: 1574
Protein: 106 g
Fat: 16 g
Sodium: 1611 mg
Cholesterol: 408 mg (without egg yolk, 143 mg)

MEAL PLAN 7

Breakfast   Call-the-Police Carrot Muffins with Applesauce
                (page 136)
Lunch   Vivacious Vegetable Pitas with Blueberries
                (page 176)
Dinner   Hot Flounder Chili Fillets with Spinach (page 221)
Snacks   Lucky Vanilla-Lemon Lift Cookies and Milk (page
                260)
                Bodybuilding Blueberry-Rum Rice Pudding (page
                277)

TOTALS FOR THE DAY
Calories: 1654
Protein: 111 g
Fat: 23 g
Sodium: 1525 mg
Cholesterol: 169 mg

MEAL PLAN 8

Breakfast   Bella Russia Potato Pancakes and Sour Cream
                (page 141)
Lunch   Kid Gloves Stand-Up Sandwich with Mixed
                Vegetables (page 180)
Dinner   Confidence Chicken Cacciatore and Peas (page
                230)

Snacks   Watermelon and Strawberries (page 248)
               Apple

TOTALS FOR THE DAY
Calories: 1758
Protein: 151 g
Fat: 17 g
Sodium: 1370 mg
Cholesterol: 196 mg

Note: Calories are high. You may cut the chicken cacciatore recipe in half.

MEAL PLAN 9

Breakfast Energy Egg Drop Soup with Kiwi (page 125)
Lunch   Pyramid Pasta Chicken Salad with Tangerines
               (page 189)
Dinner   Runner's Rice and Black Beans With Okra
               (page 240)
Snacks   Apple Jacks Candy (page 247)
               1 Baked Potato (page 126)

TOTALS FOR THE DAY
Calories: 1568
Protein: 81 g
Fat: 15 g
Sodium: 1053 mg
Cholesterol: 338 mg

MEAL PLAN 10

Breakfast Slavic Stuffed Baked Potato with Honeydew
               (page 151)
Lunch   Grandma's Old-Fashioned Mushroom Spinach
               Soup (page 192)

	Kiev Cottage Cheese and Pumpernickel Sandwich and Salad (page 156)
Dinner	Spicy Mahimahi with Brown Rice and Cauliflower (page 239)
Snacks	Raisins (page 249) and Raw Vegetable Plate (page 249)

TOTALS FOR THE DAY
Calories: 1582
Protein: 115 g
Fat: 13 g
Sodium: 1536 mg
Cholesterol: 256 mg

MEAL PLAN 11

Breakfast	Bagel and Lox Without the Lox—and with Half a Grapefruit (page 117)
Lunch	Boom-Boom Black Bean Soup (page 194) Tangy Tuna-Cucumber-Onion Sandwich on Whole Wheat with Red Peppers and Tomatoes (page 157)
Dinner	Microwave Vegetable-Flounder Stew with White Rice (page 201)
Snacks	Cinnamon-Apple Oatmeal (page 250) V-8 Juice (page 250) 1/2 cup 1% cottage cheese

TOTALS FOR THE DAY
Calories: 1388
Protein: 109 g
Fat: 15 g
Sodium: 2432 mg
Cholesterol: 155 mg

MEAL PLAN 12

Breakfast Raisin Oatmeal Rise-and-Shine Pancakes with
              Raspberries (page 145)
Lunch   Vitamin-Vixen Vegetable Salmon Sandwich
              (page 184)
Dinner   Shrimp-Vegetable Peak Contraction Pasta
              (page 238)
Snacks   Tangy Romaine-Mushroom-Mustard Salad with a
              Pear (page 273)
              Minestrone Soup (page 247)

TOTALS FOR THE DAY
Calories: 1727
Protein: 94 g
Fat: 21 g
Sodium: 1536 mg
Cholesterol: 92 mg

MEAL PLAN 13

Breakfast Blueberry Wheat Wake-Up Pancakes with
              Blueberries (page 144)
Lunch   Big-Boy Broiled Pepper and Onion Sandwich with
              Pineapple (page 183)
Dinner   Mother's Vegetable Delight with Sea Bass
              (page 235)
Snacks   Italian Vegetable Salad (page 270)
              Raspberry-Peach Milkshake (page 279)

TOTALS FOR THE DAY
Calories: 1431
Protein: 118 g
Fat: 13 g
Sodium: 1818 mg
Cholesterol: 201 mg

MEAL PLAN 14

Breakfast Busy Bee Banana-Strawberry Pancakes with Sliced
Strawberries (page 142)
Lunch Cutting-Edge Egg White Sandwich and Broccoli
(page 181)
Dinner Hungry Woman's Halibut, Brown Rice, and Carrots
(page 231)
Snacks Energizing Eggplant-Tomato-Mushroom Bake
(page 268)
1 cup raspberries
Red-Eye Mashed Potatoes (page 266)

TOTALS FOR THE DAY
Calories: 1705
Protein: 111 g
Fat: 18 g
Sodium: 1293 mg
Cholesterol: 95 mg

MEAL PLAN 15

Breakfast Barbell Banana-Almond-Raisin Muffins with Sliced
Banana (page 137)
Lunch All-in-One Lunch: Tofu–Fresh Vegetable Pita
Delight (page 177)
Dinner Titanium Woman's Turkey Cutlets and Linguine
with Cucumbers and Tomatoes (page 222)
Snacks Joyce's Peppy Potato Salad (page 266)
Preconditioning Cherry-Rice Bake (page 275)

TOTALS FOR THE DAY
Calories: 1668
Protein: 106 g
Fat: 14 g
Sodium: 1129 mg
Cholesterol: 148 mg

MEAL PLAN 16

Breakfast Pineapple Perk-Up Muffins with Pineapple Chunks (page 138)
Lunch Luscious Lettuce and Tomato Sandwich with Vegetables (page 158)
Dinner Broiled Flounder and Tomatoes, Mushrooms, and Onions with Broccoli and Fried Brown Rice (page 207)
Snacks Sinful Sweet Potato Slices (page 267)
Self-Confidence Caesar Salad (page 271)

TOTALS FOR THE DAY
Calories: 1609
Protein: 99 g
Fat: 16 g
Sodium: 1477 mg
Cholesterol: 142 mg

MEAL PLAN 17

Breakfast Cold Cereal Quickie with Strawberries (page 121)
Lunch Turkey Trot on Toast with Green Beans (page 164)
Dinner Pasta with Vegetables and Springtime Salad (page 212)
Snacks Egg White Sandwich (page 250)
Accent on Asparagus Pea Soup (page 196)

TOTALS FOR THE DAY
Calories: 1316
Protein: 94 g
Fat: 15 g
Sodium: 1343 mg
Cholesterol: 78 mg

MEAL PLAN 18

Breakfast   Joyce's Red, White, and Blue Delight
(page 124)
Lunch   Yogurt and Fruit Fiesta with English Bran Muffin
and Milk (page 161)
Dinner   Sweet-and-Sour Tofu Mini-Burgers with Brown
Rice and Broccoli (page 225)
Snacks   Rice Cakes (page 252)
Lettuce and Tomato Salad (page 256)

TOTALS FOR THE DAY
Calories: 1578
Protein: 75 g
Fat: 23 g
Sodium: 1219 mg
Cholesterol: 152 mg

MEAL PLAN 19

Breakfast   Popeye's Wake-Up Pizza with Papaya
(page 149)
Lunch   Top Shape Turkey-Apricot Salad with Wheat Germ
(page 188)
Dinner   Squid-Squeeze Fettuccine with Mushrooms and
Tomatoes (page 232)
Snacks   Broccoli and Cauliflower (page 249)
1 cup raspberries
Angel Food Cake or Cupcakes (page 253)

TOTALS FOR THE DAY
Calories: 1302
Protein: 100 g
Fat: 22 g
Sodium: 515 mg
Cholesterol: 235 mg

MEAL PLAN 20

Breakfast   Jumping Gingerbread-Nutmeg Apple Pancakes
with Apples (page 146)
Glass of 1% milk

Lunch   Bodybuilder's Brown Rice and Chicken Salad
(page 186)

Dinner   Leg-Curl Eggplant Lasagne with Carrots,
Asparagus, and Salad (page 228)

Snacks   Jerusalem Artichokes (page 255)
Time-Out Tomato-Mushroom Snack (page 274)
1/4 honeydew melon

TOTALS FOR THE DAY
Calories: 1693
Protein: 140 g
Fat: 21 g
Sodium: 2189 mg
Cholesterol: 156 mg

MEAL PLAN 21

Breakfast   Three Little Bears on-the-Run Porridge with Pear
(page 119)

Lunch   Happy Heart Carrot-Squash Soup (page 193)
Self-Esteem Sea Bass and Brown Rice Salad
(page 190)

Dinner   Tossed Tofu Dinner in a Salad with Pita Bread and
Grapefruit (page 203)

Snacks   Popcorn (page 251)
Strut-Your-Stuff Green Bean Patties (page 274)

TOTALS FOR THE DAY
Calories: 1593
Protein: 94 g
Fat: 22 g
Sodium: 2532 mg
Cholesterol: 65 mg

MEAL PLAN 22

Breakfast Banana-Boat Beauty Queen (page 118) without
toast
Bagel and Cream Cheese (page 246) without plums
Lunch Strongman's Tangy Tuna (page 179)
Dinner Microwave Dill-Sole Stew with Brown Rice
(page 202)
Snacks Pretzels (page 251)
Peas and Carrots (page 252)

TOTALS FOR THE DAY
Calories: 1717
Protein: 130 g
Fat: 14 g
Sodium: 2655 mg
Cholesterol: 192 mg

MEAL PLAN 23

Breakfast Buckeye Opener Pancakes with Apricots
(page 143)
Glass of 1% milk
Lunch Turkey-Trot Sandwich and Cauliflower (page 182)
Dinner Barbara's Bull's-Eye Rice and Beans (page 234)
Snacks Succulent Sautéed Soy Vegetables and Swordfish
(page 269)
Winter Squash and Broccoli Steambath
(page 270)
1 cup raspberries

TOTALS FOR THE DAY
Calories: 1518
Protein: 97 g
Fat: 17 g
Sodium: 2941 mg
Cholesterol: 138 mg

MEAL PLAN 24

Breakfast Aerobic Bran-Apple Muffins with Stuffed Apple
              (page 140)
Lunch   Chicken and Brown Rice Mushroom Madness
              (page 178)
Dinner   Protein-Power Tofu-Potatoes and Zucchini
              (page 226)
Snacks   Bagel and Cream Cheese Sweet Peach Sit-Ups
              (page 118)
              Cut-Up Carrot-Spinach Soup (page 272)

TOTALS FOR THE DAY
Calories: 1337
Protein: 87 g
Fat: 16 g
Sodium: 1237 mg
Cholesterol: 139 mg

MEAL PLAN 25

Breakfast Spicy Superset Omelet and Toast (page 131)
Lunch   Vivacious Vegetable Pizza with Asparagus
              (page 168)
Dinner   Cheeky Chicken and Brown Rice Pilaf
              (page 218)
Snacks   Apple-Pear-Peach Salad (page 277)
              Green Beans and Carrots (page 218)

TOTALS FOR THE DAY
Calories: 1621
Protein: 81 g
Fat: 15 g
Sodium: 725 mg
Cholesterol: 76 mg

MEAL PLAN 26

Breakfast Rousing Russian Potato Soup (page 194)
Lunch Flounder Patty and Brown Rice with Vegetables (page 174)
Dinner Amazing Mushroom Tofu Burgers with Tomato and Onion (page 224)
Cranberry-Cherry Cottage Cheese Pudding (page 278)
Snacks Rousing Rutabaga (page 258)
Bagel and Cream Cheese (page 246) without plums
V-8 Juice (page 250)

TOTALS FOR THE DAY
Calories: 1297
Protein: 91 g
Fat: 21 g
Sodium: 1477 mg
Cholesterol: 117 mg

MEAL PLAN 27

Breakfast Biceps Buttermilk Pancakes with Tangerines and Milk (page 147)
Lunch Luscious Lentil Lift Salad (page 187)
1 Baked Potato (page 126)
Dinner Orange-Pineapple Chicken with Brown Rice and Mushrooms (page 236)
Snacks Bagel and Cream Cheese (page 246) without plums
Corn on the Cob with Butter Buds (page 247)

TOTALS FOR THE DAY
Calories: 1551
Protein: 112 g
Fat: 15 g
Sodium: 989 mg
Cholesterol: 121 mg

MEAL PLAN 28

Breakfast   Hearty Oatmeal and Mango Day Starter
(page 120)

Lunch   Tantalizing Tuna Toss and Toast (page 160)

Dinner   Broiled Red Snapper, Red Peppers, and Onions
with Corn on the Cob (page 204)

Snacks   Beat-the-Hunger Broccoli-Cauliflower-Carrot Soup
(page 195)

1/2 grapefruit

Nonfat or Low-Fat Yogurt and 3 Low-Fat Melba
Rounds (page 127)

TOTALS FOR THE DAY
Calories: 1314 g
Protein: 116 g
Fat: 13 g
Sodium: 778 mg
Cholesterol: 127 mg

MEAL PLAN 29

Breakfast   Power Potato-Plum Energy Breakfast
(page 150)

Lunch   Gut Buster Gazpacho Soup (page 197)
Speed-Set Salmon Sandwich with Vegetables
(page 163)

Dinner   Stir-Fried Vegetables and Brown Rice with Turkey
Breast (page 211)

Snacks   Broiled Pepper, Onion, Tomato, and Mushrooms
(page 254)
Raspberry Sorbet or ice pops (page 256)

TOTALS FOR THE DAY
Calories: 1312
Protein: 90 g
Fat: 18 g
Sodium: 931 mg
Cholesterol: 111 mg

MEAL PLAN 30

Breakfast   Catch-Me-If-You-Can Cornbread Crunch with
              Cantaloupe (page 128)
Lunch   Dragon Lady's Spicy Rice and Vegetables
              (page 166)
Dinner   Joyce's Security Blanket Chicken Soup and Rice
              (page 214)
Snacks   Mango-Strawberry Delight (page 279)
              Baked Athletic Cinnamon-Raisin Squash with
              Cottage Cheese (page 257)

TOTALS FOR THE DAY
Calories: 1604
Protein: 121 g
Fat: 14 g
Sodium: 1583 mg
Cholesterol: 202 mg

MEAL PLAN 31

Breakfast   English Muffin Motivation with Grapes
              (page 122)
Lunch   End-All Egg Salad Sandwich with Stir-Fried
              Vegetables (page 165)
Dinner   Marinated Chicken and Orzo (page 206)
              1 cup cauliflower
Snacks   Pickle-Pepper Salad (page 256)
              Baked Sweet Potato (page 254)
              2 small kiwi fruit

TOTALS FOR THE DAY
Calories: 1327
Protein: 90 g
Fat: 15 g
Sodium: 1942 mg
Cholesterol: 370 mg (without egg yolk, 105)

WHEN YOU'RE AWAY FROM HOME

You can now plan your meals at home and keep to your healthy, low-fat eating plan without a problem. But what do you do when you're eating out? Or worse, when you're away on a vacation or a business trip, when you have to eat out for days or even weeks at a time? And what do you do on the plane going and coming? When you've been invited to someone's home for dinner? Finally, what do you do when you're away from home all day but are so busy that you just won't have time to stop in a restaurant and sit down for a meal?

In the following paragraphs you'll find out how to get a grip on such situations.

In a Restaurant

Thankfully, restaurant dining has become easier because many establishments now have the calorie and fat content posted right on the "Healthy Eating" (or similar) section of the menu. If this is the case, no problem. You simply choose the dish lowest in fat and calories that suits you. But what if no such menu exists? Most of the time you can get a food item if you ask for it, especially if it's a staple item. Let's take one meal at a time.

Breakfast. You can always have two slices of whole wheat toast and a teaspoon or even a tablespoon of regular jam or jelly. If you want to forgo the jelly, you can ask for a sliced tomato and some lettuce, and make a little sandwich, flavoring it a bit with some wine vinegar.

Most restaurants have English muffins or bagels; you could have a half or even a whole of either. If it's a bagel, ask for nonfat cream cheese. If they don't have that, use jam or jelly or the tomatoes and lettuce. Or you could have a poached egg on two slices of whole wheat toast—as long as you haven't had more than two eggs that week and you take into account the fat grams. What about butter or margarine? No. They are too high in fat while you're trying to lose weight.

Another idea for breakfast is oatmeal. You can't really lose there, as long as you don't load it with full-fat milk and sugar. I put salt in my oatmeal and no milk—and I also love Tabasco sauce. I learned this secret when I was a guest at The Pritikin Longevity Center in Miami, Florida. Wow, does it kick up the oatmeal! Don't worry about what the waiter or waitress thinks—just ask for the sauce. After all, it's your butt or thighs that will have the extra lard covering them—and where will those people be to help you when that happens?

And then there's always cold cereal, but only if they have 1 percent milk or skim milk. You could ask for the fruit in season (berries, for example) and put them in the cereal.

Lunch. Soup is always a good bet, as long as it isn't a cream variety. Chicken with rice or chicken noodle, vegetable, minestrone, tomato—there are loads of acceptable soups. You can have the soup with a large tossed salad and dress it with some balsamic or wine vinegar. You can have half a grapefruit or cantaloupe on the side. Keep in mind that soup is often high in sodium. You may retain water, but don't worry—unless you have high blood pressure or other health issues that require you to be careful about sodium. The weight gain is temporary and will not make you fat. I eat soup all the time—full sodium or partially reduced sodium—and I love it.

Another idea is to ask if the restaurant has tuna packed in water, and order it on a bed of lettuce surrounded with tomatoes. You can even ask for two slices of whole wheat bread and make it into a sandwich. If they don't have whole wheat bread, order pumpernickel or rye or any other whole-grain bread. If they don't have anything but white bread, you can have that.

You may be in the mood for a large fruit salad, which is often served with low-fat yogurt. In my experience, you can forget about getting nonfat yogurt in a restaurant. Don't worry; the low-fat is good enough. Sometimes they serve the fruit salad with cottage cheese, but be careful. It's usually full-fat cottage cheese (4 percent—too much fat). Ask for low or non-fat cottage cheese. If they don't have it, skip the cottage cheese.

Finally, there's the salad bar. You can have lettuce, tomatoes, beans of all kinds (as long as they're not in anything oily), vegetables (usually green beans, beets, carrots). These days most salad bars have nonfat dressings, so you can really go to town. If they don't, ask for wine or balsamic vinegar—or even plain white vinegar. You can even have the pickles, if you don't mind the high sodium. (I can eat a whole jar of pickles over a day's time, but I have very low blood pressure. I sometimes think that's why my body craves sodium. You do what's best for you.)

Sandwiches are a great choice for lunch. The best idea is a white-meat turkey sandwich, but ask if the meat is cut fresh from the turkey; otherwise, it will be the high-sodium processed kind—not as tasty and causes you to retain water. You can put tomatoes, lettuce, and mustard on the sandwich. Sometimes there's a vegetarian pita filled with all sorts of delicious vegetables and sprouts. This is great as long as the dressing is on the side. It's usually high in fat, so skip it and ask for nonfat dressing or the vinegars discussed above.

Dinner. The best deal in town when it comes to dinner out is broiled fish. But pick a low-fat fish and make sure the cook does not brush it with olive oil (they foolishly try to convince you that it's okay because it's olive oil, but you know that olive oil makes you just as fat). Choose flounder, sole, or mahimahi as first choices—they are very low in fat. You can have any vegetables on the side, but make sure they are not cooked with butter. If they come looking buttery, throw them into a napkin and blot them to death. You can have a plain baked potato on the side and eat it with a wedge of lemon and pepper and salt, or you can put a little ketchup on the potato.

Instead of fish, you can have broiled chicken breast (remove the skin) or a few slices of turkey breast, with vegetables prepared with no butter and a baked potato on the side. If you don't like the potato, ask for plain white or brown rice. Believe it or not, you can usually get white rice—with nothing on it—in any restaurant if you insist.

Another dinner idea is pasta, but be sure to order marinara or other tomato sauce without meat. Also ask if the marinara is cooked with a lot of oil. Very often they lie to you outright, and when the pasta arrives you can see the oil. If this happens, send it back.

One of my favorite pasta dishes is a mixture of seafood and pasta in a tomato sauce, called seafood fra diablo. The shrimp and clams are high in cholesterol, but it's not the artery-clogging cholesterol (as in fat). (Doctors agree that if your cholesterol is high, just to be on the safe side you must keep all cholesterol down, even the low-fat cholesterol found in seafood.)

A chef's salad is always a good bet, but if and only if they hold the cheese and roast beef, and double up the white meat turkey or chicken. You can let them leave the eggs in, but eat only the whites. If you have the salad with nonfat dressing or wine or balsamic vinegar, it's quite tasty.

Many times the lunch menu overlaps the dinner menu, so anything I say for dinner can apply to lunch. In fact, if you can get it, you can eat a breakfast food for lunch or dinner. Who cares?

What about room service? In most hotels, the all-day dining menu is the same as the foods listed on the regular menu, only the fancy foods are not available. Those are the elaborate fatty dinners that you wouldn't choose anyway. For example, you can always get a tossed or chef's salad, whole wheat toast, a fruit salad, soup, and so on.

On the Airplane

Thankfully, if you think ahead (up to twenty-four hours before flight time), all major airlines will order you a low-fat meal. Depending upon their meal titles, order either a low-fat or low-calorie meal. If neither of these are available, order a vegetarian meal, but beware that such meals could be high in oil or other fat.

But what if you forgot to order a special meal, or—as happens all too often—your special meal just doesn't turn up? You usually get a choice of meals. For breakfast, choose the cold cereal and fruit over the fatty French toast or cheese omelet. For lunch or dinner, choose the fish or chicken over the beef—and then blot each food item until the excess fat is gone. Don't forget to blot the vegetables; they're usually loaded with butter or oil.

For a drink, have either club soda or a diet drink, or coffee or tea with skim or 1 percent milk. Many airlines now carry low-fat milk.

If you really want to be sure to keep your eating low in fat on a plane, bring your own food. A can of tuna packed in water and a couple slices of whole wheat bread, along with a tomato and a piece of fruit, will do the trick just fine. You can use this in an emergency, if you see that the meal being served is hopelessly full of fat. Better safe than sorry. After all, why spoil all your hard work just because the airline isn't playing your game?

At Someone's Home

Suppose you're doing great on your diet, and then in the middle of it you have to attend a dinner and you just know that it's going to blow the whole thing. You have to make a decision: Is it worth giving up your hard work just to avoid the discomfort of asking the host or hostess to help you?

If the answer is no, call the host or hostess *ahead of time* and tell of your predicament. I've even asked if I could bring a piece of chicken (to work around the offered vegetables). Often the host or hostess insists on broiling me a piece of chicken or fish. I can then eat the vegetables and salad—no problem.

The only other option is to simply eat only what is low in fat—and plenty of it. If someone comments on your not eating the main dish, you say you have a sensitive stomach and are under a doctor's care. (I have friends who can eat almost nothing owing to irritable bowel syndrome, for example.)

At a Buffet-Style Business Meeting

Business meetings are affairs that seem quite safe on the surface, but can sabotage your diet without your even realizing it. There is usually food of every kind, spread out on various tables: plates full of ham, roast beef, leg of lamb, pork, meatballs, all sorts of pastas and greasy salads—you name it.

But if you take a closer look, you will also notice some edible foods: loads of fresh shrimp, white meat chicken or turkey, delicious tomatoes, cucumbers, radishes, and carrots, and lots of fresh fruit. There's no reason why you can't keep to your low-fat eating plan with ease in such a situation.

If this is true, then why do so many people blow their diet on such occasions? The answer is quite simple. We "pick," and we do it almost unconsciously. We sidle up to the table and just sneak a piece of this or that—just to taste it, of course. Then we circle around another table and snap up another harmless morsel. We do this a few more times, and before you know it, we say to ourselves, "It's not every day I get to have such deliciously prepared food. There's mountains of it. What a waste. What harm will there be if I just eat what I want this one time?"

That's it. The end of your low-fat eating for that day. But it doesn't have to be that way. If you prepare yourself mentally before the banquet, and employ the preconditioning and visualization techniques mentioned in Chapter 2, you can head off trouble before it starts.

When You Don't Have Time to Stop for a Meal

I've already told you what to do when you're leaving your house in a rush and don't have time for breakfast. But what do you do when you're already out and you've brought no food with you, and you simply don't have time to sit down in a restaurant for a meal? We'll take it one meal at a time.

For breakfast, purchase a nonfat yogurt or cottage cheese, whole wheat bread, and a piece of fruit and bring them to the office or eat them in the car. You can buy plastic forks if the establishment doesn't have them to give away.

For lunch, you can get a white meat turkey sandwich if you have the time to wait until it is made up. Otherwise, you can buy a can of tuna packed in water—with the pull-off top so you don't have to use a can opener. Get a couple of tomatoes and a cucumber, a couple of red peppers and a piece of fruit. You can eat this in the car or in the office.

For dinner, do the same as lunch, or get a couple of slices of pizza on the run. You can ask for little or no cheese. Some places have fat-free pizza, whole wheat pizza with fresh vegetables, and so on. There may be endless choices. In any case, if the pizza has oil, cheese, or fat of any kind on it, you can blot it with a few napkins.

For snacks, buy a bagel or soft pretzel—and even eat it walking to a destination. You can drink bottled water or diet soda, or some juice and a piece of fruit or two.

There's no reason—no excuse—to throw your diet out the window just because you have no time to eat. You can and must eat—preferably five times a day—no matter where you are or what you're doing. You can mix and match, and space it out any way you want. But even if you're away from home all day, without a minute to sit down to a meal in a restaurant, you can get some food and feed it to your body—the machine that keeps you going. You can do it if you realize how important it is to keep losing weight and being healthy—and prevent you from binging and gaining back the weight (because that's just what happens when you starve yourself all day).

Another reason to eat five times a day is to keep your metabolism moving. When you deprive your body of food for more than four to five hours, your metabolism slows down and you burn fewer calories than you would if you had a light meal. The body goes into a survival mechanism—it begins to save energy in defense of what it perceives of as an upcoming famine. So it's much better to eat more often—light meals—than to wait all day and eat one big meal. In the long run, you burn more fat.

WORKING AROUND A FAMILY WHO IS *NOT* DIETING

I'll say it up front: It's not easy! If your husband loves fried foods and calls himself a "meat and potatoes man," or your teens demand fat-filled deserts and even bring them into the house in spite of your protest, what can you do?

It's a real test of willpower. First, you have remind yourself that there is no way the fatty foods can get into your mouth unless you put them there. That is to say, cooking and serving does not make you fat—but tasting does. This may be the time to put the tape over your mouth when you're cooking, an idea mentioned in Chapter 4. I was kidding but not kidding when I said it.

But you won't have to do that if you have a talk with yourself. "I can cook this pork loin, but I don't have to eat it," you can say. And to help yourself, cook your own meal first, and then have some unlimited vegetables on the side in a bowl as you cook. Instead of nibbling on the fatty food, nibble on the red peppers in vinegar or the cucumbers. It works, but only if you want it to work.

But what about cooking two separate meals? I'll admit it. It's a hassle. It's extra work. Who needs it? Well, you do. Unless you can convince the rest of your family to join your low-fat eating plan, there's no other way. And when you weigh the benefits against the effort, it's *really* worth it. Do what you have to do. Cook ahead. Freeze the foods. Survive. It's your life. It's your peace of mind. No one is going to do it for you! Don't let anything stop you. You can do it.

WORKING AROUND A LIMITED FOOD BUDGET

You put in the extra effort. You're willing to cook separate meals, but what if your food budget is very limited? You're used to buying what's on sale—fat or no fat.

You can look for vegetable and fruit sales. And instead of eating the more expensive low-fat white meat chicken, turkey, and fish—which could cost a good bundle—stick to beans. I recently discovered rice and beans. I buy all the Goya beans and mix them with rice. Wow! How filling, how inexpensive, how low in fat, how filled with nutrition, and how delicious. Small white beans, small red beans, white or red kidney beans, black beans, black-eyed peas, and on and on. (If you rinse the canned beans, you reduce the sodium content by 40 percent.)

Go to town. Look at all the calculations on the cans, or better, since they're less expensive, buy packages of dried beans and make them up yourself. You could live on rice and beans for a year (of course, you would want to add vegetables and fruit). I eat at least two servings of beans with two servings of rice for a meal, and am still well within the calorie and fat allowances for the day. In fact, vegetarians who eat mainly rice and beans for their protein are usually much thinner than meat eaters—and I mean even poultry and fish eaters.

NOTHING CAN STOP YOU

The power is yours! When it comes right down to it, thank God, the truth is that no one is force-feeding us. If anything goes into our mouths, it's because we put it there. We reach down and pick up the fork or spoon, and we put some food on it. We raise the utensil to our mouths, moving it from point A to point B. We then chew the food and swallow it. Again and again, we go through this motion until X amount of food is consumed. And if what we've eaten is not in tune with our weight-loss program, we mercilessly berate ourselves for not having self-control.

It's time to stop beating up on yourself and, at the same time, brainwashing yourself to believe that you can't help yourself. You've gained weight because you've developed some bad habits when it comes to food. Now you can change those habits—not by depriving yourself and not eating when you're hungry, but by changing what you eat when you're hungry. That way, when the eating session is over, no damage has been done.

This is a new day in your life. You can change your body

gradually, as you learn to stop eating to your chagrin (the wrong foods) and start eating to trim (the foods outlined in this book). And whenever you get discouraged, think of me. I'm right there with you, feeling the same way you do about food. I love it. But I've learned to control it—it no longer controls me. And you can do the same.

I'd love to hear how you're doing. Write to me at the address on page 344. If you enclose a stamped, self-addressed envelope, I'll personally answer your letter.

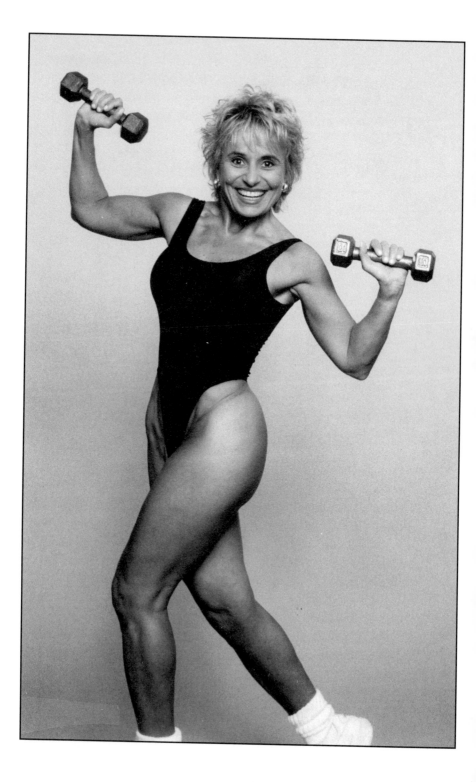

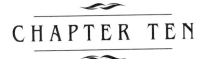

CHAPTER TEN

WHAT ABOUT EXERCISE?

Without exercise, the diet is often—no, usually—in vain. It's an endless merry-go-round! If you diet and don't exercise, it will be only a matter of time before you gain back the weight you lost.

So you must exercise. But how? Not just any exercise will do. To ensure that you keep the weight off, you must do a specific kind of exercise—exercise that will permanently raise your metabolism so that you can eat more than you used to eat without getting fat. According to studies cited in "Strength Training Update," working out 8 to 12 weeks adds about 3 pounds of lean muscle and raises the metabolic rate by about 7 percent and the daily calorie requirement by 15 percent. "Adults who add muscle through sensible strength exercise use more calories all day long, so are less likely to accumulate fat," says Wayne L. Prescott, Ph.D.[1]

1. Wayne L. Prescott, Ph.D., "Strength Training Update," *Idea Today* (June 1995), p. 1.

The kind of exercise I'm talking about makes your body a permanent fat-burning furnace so that you burn more fat twenty-four hours a day, even while you're sleeping. In fact, after working out, as described in this chapter, for even twelve weeks, you can eat about 15 percent more than you did without gaining weight.

But what is this right exercise? If you have any of my workout books, or have heard me on television, you already know what I'm going to say. You must work out with weights so that you can place mini-muscles all over your body. Now don't panic; I'm not talking the "Arnold" kind of weight lifting. Since muscle is the only body material that is active twenty-four hours a day (blood, water, bone, skin, and fat are all stagnant), you burn more calories and you lose more weight.

MUSCLES GIVE YOU SHAPE

I never had a great shape. Even at twenty-four, when I wasn't fat, I didn't look good. My shoulders were sloped downward, my hips were wide, and my legs were misshapen. (There's a photograph of me on page 11 of *Bottoms Up!* to prove this point.) I was not lucky when it came to genetics, not to mention the fact that I'm not quite five feet tall. So for me, weights were a miracle. They enabled me to not only put fat-burning muscle on my body but also to sculpt the perfect body. That's why now, at fifty-three, I can honestly say I have a better shape than I did when I was half my age.

But guess what? Even women who have perfect genetics and *never got fat*, who are my age or even as young as forty, now no longer have great shapes. Why? Because every year after thirty, a half pound of muscle atrophies, so that eventually even if you are not overweight, your skin hangs over your kneecaps and your arms wave like flags in the wind. In fact, your entire body feels soft rather than toned. This is the result of normal muscle atrophy. But thankfully you can change all that—and the remedy is not that difficult. You *must* (and there is no choice here, it's a *must*) work out with weights in a specific manner to put muscle in all the right places to fill out that sagging skin, so that once again you can feel firm and look great.

Not only will working with weights reshape your body and give you the figure you never had, it will also increase your bone density and reverse osteoporosis. Even though I've been through menopause, my bone is nearly double the density of women my age who do not work out with weights. Study after study shows that working with weights even for twelve weeks significantly raises the metabolism by 15 percent, so that you can eat more without getting fat.

What About Aerobics?

Aerobics are exercises that engage the larger muscles of your body and cause your pulse to reach a rate of 60 to 80 percent of its capacity, and to stay that way for a given length of time. Experts vary in their opinion of the minimum duration exercise must be to be considered aerobic—anywhere from ten to twenty minutes, up to a maximum of an hour.

Aerobics are great for heart and lung conditioning, and they help to burn overall body fat. However, aerobics can never reshape your entire body. Swimmers have impressive backs. Soccer players have majestic legs. Tennis players have magnificent forearms—or at least one great forearm. The only way to sculpt your entire body is to work out with weights—the right way.

In addition to this workout, I encourage you to engage in your favorite aerobic activity, such as stair-stepping, brisk walking, jogging, or the exercise bike. You can do your aerobics three to six days a week, twenty to forty minutes or more. That's up to you. You can do your aerobics before or after your weight training (better before for energy) or on days you don't weight-train. But no matter what, do your weight training. That's your first priority when it comes to exercise. (Note: You can also combine weight training and aerobics, especially with my book *Definition*. I talk about choices of various workouts on pages 340 to 344.)

What Is the Right Way to Work with Weights?

The right way to work with weights is the way that will get you a double whammy: the health benefits and a perfectly sculpted body. The health benefits—replaced muscle and bone, added energy and strength, lowered blood pressure and cholesterol levels, improved posture, increased metabolism—and even a better outlook on life come with weight training.

In order to get the perfectly sculpted body, you need an expert in body sculpting—and I am that expert because I learned all my secrets from the kings and queens of all body-shaping experts—bodybuilders. It's their life. They took years to perfect the science. But most of us are afraid of bodybuilders because we don't want to look as big and hulky as they look. But we should listen to what they have to say. Why reinvent the wheel? I've taken their techniques and culled the method out of the madness (madness being creating bulk). Let me explain.

In writing for *Muscle and Fitness* magazine, over the years I've interviewed hundreds of champion bodybuilders—both male and female—and I've attended bodybuilding contests where I've seen entrants lose just because they didn't have a perfectly sculpted thigh or butt, etcetera. I've interviewed those people a few months later, when they achieved that perfectly formed body part. How did they do it? They used weights in exactly the right manner to create that shape.

How Long Does It Take to Get in Shape?

I have learned the methods of using weights and applied them to myself and others—using less weight and investing less time—and the end result is a perfectly formed "mini-body" with small sensual toning muscles in all the right places. In the following pages I show you how to get your ideal body. In three months, your body shape will have changed and you'll begin to see a lean, symmetrical figure in the mirror. In six months, you'll look nearly perfect. And as time goes on, you'll get better and better. And the best part is, you'll need to invest only *twenty minutes a day* (or less; see descriptions on pages 340 to 344, and Bibliography). That's it.

HOW TO DO THE WORKOUT

I give you a very simple workout here, but before I do you'll want to become familiar with a few basic terms that will enable you to understand the language of working out and the exercise instructions that follow.

- An *exercise* is a specific movement for a given muscle, designed to cause that muscle to do work and to become stronger and more dense, and to change shape. For example, the bench press presented in this workout is an exercise designed to shape and sculpt the chest muscles.
- A *repetition*, or a "rep," is a complete movement of an exercise, from start to midpoint to endpoint. For example, one repetition of the bench press involves raising the dumbbells from the chest position to the arms in a fully extended position, and back down to the chest position.
- A *set* is a specific number of repetitions of a given exercise that are performed without a rest. In this workout you will perform *ten repetitions* of each exercise before you take a rest.
- A *rest* is a pause between sets or exercises. The reason for resting is to allow time for your working muscle to regain enough energy to handle the next set of exercises. In this workout, you will rest *fifteen seconds* after each set. If you were using heavy weights, you would need more rest time between sets—30 seconds or more, depending upon how heavy. Bodybuilders rest from 60 to 90 seconds after each set because they use very heavy weights.

- A *routine* is the specific combination of exercises prescribed for a certain body part. For example, in this workout, your chest routine will consist of the bench press, the incline press, and the decline press.
- A *split routine* is the exercising of one half of the body one workout day and the other half of the body on the next workout day, and then back to the first half the next workout day, and so on. (You alternate—the next time you work out, you always do what you *did not do* the last time. It's that simple.) This method was invented so that people who want to work out two days in a row can do so without exhausting the muscles. (One should rest the muscles for forty-eight hours after a workout to prevent overtraining. The only exception to this rule is the abdominals and sometimes the hip/buttocks and thighs.)
- A *workout* is your entire exercise regime for a given day. For example, in this workout you will do your chest, shoulders, biceps, triceps, and back on workout day 1. That is your upper body workout. On workout day 2, you will do your thighs, hip/buttocks, abdominals, and calves. That is your lower body workout.
- *Dumbbells* are handheld weights. They are the most convenient and inexpensive of all weights and will be used for this workout instead of expensive machines. In addition, on the whole, dumbbells are more effective in body shaping than machines.

There are also some expressions I use in the exercise instructions that need to be defined. For example, I continually ask you to *flex* your working muscle and to feel the *stretch* in the muscle. You flex your muscle by squeezing it together. In essence, you temporarily shorten the muscle fibers. For example, when a person shows off his or her biceps and "makes a muscle," the biceps muscle bulges because the muscle fibers are squeezed together—the muscle is flexed. That same muscle is stretched when the person straightens out his or her arm because at this point, the muscle fibers are elongated. In this position, the muscle no longer bulges. Try it on your own biceps and see what I mean.

Sets, Repetitions, Rests, Workout Days: How to Do This Workout

I keep this workout very simple. You will do the same number of sets and repetitions and rests for each exercise: *three sets of ten repetitions*, then you *rest fifteen seconds*. It's that simple. I'll even remind you in each exercise instruction.

I give you one photo illustration for an exercise for each body part. The other two exercises you will do will be slight variations or a repeat of the first exercise. Read the instructions and you will see exactly what to do.

You will work out a minimum of *four days* a week and a maximum of *six days* a week. It's your choice. The key is that you will work half the body one day and the other half the next. You don't have to remember much when it comes to this method. All you have to remember is that you never work the same half of the body two days in a row. When you take a day off from working out, start with the half of the body you *did not work* the last time. To ensure that you won't forget, mark on your calendar "upper, lower, upper, etc." each time you work out. (You'll be surprised how easy it is to drive yourself crazy trying to remember—write it down.)

You can use a bench, or a "step" in place of a bench, for the exercises that require it. I use a step to demonstrate for those of you who may not care to invest in a bench or who may not have the space for a bench.

Which Weights Should You Use to Start?

Start with 3-pound dumbbells. (When I say 3 pounds, I mean each.) After a week or two, you will be strong enough to advance to 5-pound weights. Stay there for a while, and when you get stronger, advance to 8- or 10-pound dumbbells.

Some Body Parts Are Stronger Than Others

In advancing your weights, you will probably find that your chest, biceps, back, and thighs are strong enough to advance faster than your shoulders and triceps. If you wish, you can advance in these body parts and keep the lower weights for your weaker body parts—or you can wait until all your body parts are ready to advance. Of course, it is better to advance the body parts that are ready rather than hold them back, but that's up to you. You may not feel like investing in heavier dumbbells until your entire body demands the increase.

How Heavy Should You Go?

How long will you continue to raise your weights? Will you keep going and going until you are lifting hundreds of pounds? No! As you get stronger you can go up until you reach what I call your plateau. You'll know you are there when you are happy with the tone and look of your body. You will reach your plateau after working out for about a year. Some women go as high as 10 pounds while others go as high as 20 pounds. Perhaps you will be somewhere in the middle.

One more thing. You will not be using any weights for your stomach or hip/butt work. These body parts don't need weights because of the nature of their makeup—you don't want bulky abs or a bigger butt!

Breaking in Gently

Unless you are already a seasoned weight trainer (you've done a regular weight workout consistently in the past), follow this break-in-gently system.

Week 1. Do the entire workout with no weights—just do the movements.

Week 2. Do only one set of each exercise for the entire workout (using weights from now on).

Week 3. Do only two sets of each exercise for the entire workout.

Week 4. Do three sets of each exercise. You are now doing the complete workout.

Note: Whenever I say "bench" you may substitute "step" if you wish.

WORKOUT DAY 1 UPPER BODY WORKOUT

Chest: Flat Dumbbell Press and Incline Dumbbell Press

Develops, shapes, strengthens, and defines the entire chest (pectoral) area.

Exercise 1

Position: Lie on a flat exercise bench with a dumbbell held in each hand, palms facing upward, and with the outer edge of the dumbbells touching your upper chest area.

Movement: Flexing your chest muscles as you go, extend your arms upward until your elbows are nearly locked. The dumbbells should be in line with your upper chest in this fully extended position. Willfully flex your chest muscles and return to start position. Feel the stretch in your chest muscles and repeat the movement until you have completed your set.

Rest 15 seconds and perform your second set of this exercise. Rest another 15 seconds and perform your third and last set of this exercise.

Now move to the next exercise in your chest routine—the incline dumbbell press—and again do three sets as you did here. Then move to the final exercise in your chest routine—a repeat of the first exercise, the flat dumbbell press—and again do three sets of this exercise. Then move to your next body part, shoulders.

Note: You do the incline dumbbell press exactly the same way as the flat dumbbell press, only you raise the step to an incline by adding an additional piece (about 8 inches, supplied with the step) to one side of the step. You place your head on the incline.

Beware: In order to get a full stretch in your chest, be sure to extend your elbows fully downward on the down movement. Keep your mind focused on your chest muscles throughout the exercise.

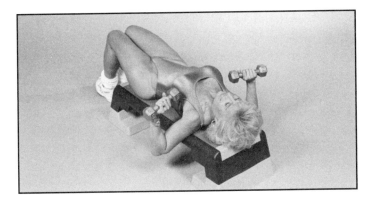

Start

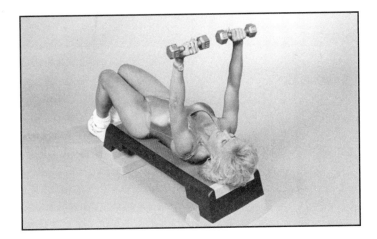

Finish

Exercise 2: Perform the same movement on an incline (5–10 inches).

Note: For incline, raise the step by removing one of the plastic blocks and lying on the appropriate end.

Exercise 3: Repeat the first exercise in this routine, the flat dumbbell press.

Sets, Repetitions, Weights: Do three sets of 10 repetitions each. Rest 15 seconds between each set. Use 3-pound dumbbells and go higher as you get stronger.

Shoulders: Alternate Shoulder Press and Double-Arm Shoulder Press

Develops, shapes, strengthens, and defines entire shoulder muscle, especially the front area of this muscle.

Exercise 1

Position: Stand with your feet together or in a natural position, holding a dumbbell in each hand at shoulder height, with your palms facing away from your body.

Movement: Raise your right arm upward until it is fully extended. While returning your right arm to the start position, begin raising your left arm upward until it is fully extended, while at the same time lowering your right arm. Continue this alternate up-and-down movement until you have completed your set.

Rest 15 seconds and perform your second set of this exercise. Rest another 15 seconds and perform your third and last set of this exercise.

Now move to the next exercise in your shoulder routine, the double-arm shoulder press. (Perform this exercise in exactly the same manner, only do both arms at the same time.) Again do three sets as you did here. Then move to the final exercise in your shoulder routine, a repeat of the first exercise, the alternate shoulder press, and again do three sets of this exercise. Then move to your next body part, biceps.

Beware: Keep your upper body steady as you work. Remember to flex your shoulder muscle on each upward movement and to feel the stretch on each down position.

Exercise 2: Perform the same movement two arms at a time.

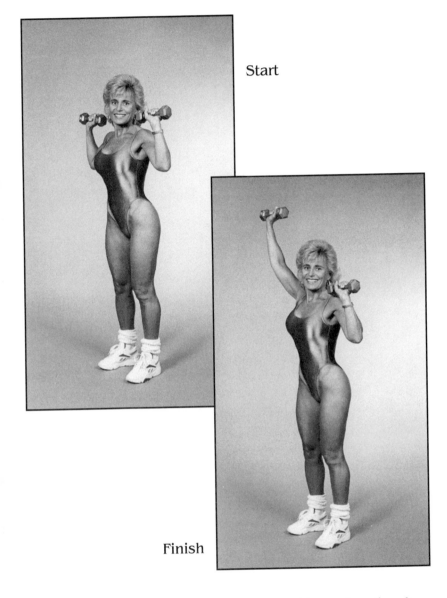

Start

Finish

Exercise 3:   Repeat the first exercise in this routine, the alternate shoulder press.

Sets, Repetitions, Weights: Do three sets of 10 repetitions each. Rest 15 seconds between each set. Use 3-pound dumbbells and go higher as you get stronger.

Biceps: Simultaneous Standing Curl, Alternate Biceps Curl, Alternate Hammer Curl

Develops, shapes, strengthens, and defines the entire biceps muscle and helps to strengthen the forearm.

Exercise 1

Position: Stand with your feet together or a natural width apart with a dumbbell in each hand. Place your arms at your sides and hold the dumbbells palms facing your body.

Movement: Flexing your biceps muscles as you go and keeping your arms close to your body and your wrists slightly curled upward, rotate your wrists and curl your arms upward simultaneously until you cannot curl them any further. Willfully flex your biceps muscles and return to start position. Feel the stretch in your biceps muscles and repeat the movement until you have completed your set.

Rest 15 seconds and perform your second set of this exercise. Rest another 15 seconds and perform your third and last set of this exercise.

Now move to the next exercise in your biceps routine, the alternate biceps curl. (Perform this exercise exactly the same way as the simultaneous standing curl, only do one arm at a time.) Again do three sets as you did here. Then move to the final exercise in your biceps routine, the alternate hammer curl. (Perform this exercise in exatly the same way as the alternate biceps curl, only hold the dumbbells in a hammerlike position, palms facing your body.) Again do three sets of this exercise. Then move to your next body part, triceps.

Beware: Don't rock back and forth as you work. Your body should remain stationary—only your arms are

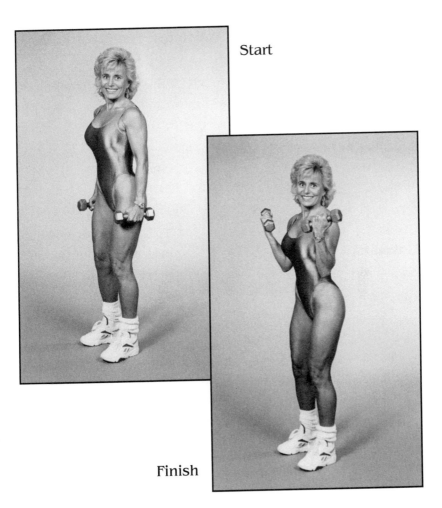

Start

Finish

moving. Don't hold your breath. Breathe naturally.

Exercise 2: Perform this exercise one arm at a time (alternate biceps curl).

Exercise 3: Perform this exercise one arm at a time in the "hammer" position (alternate hammer curl.) Turn the dumbbells facing your body and "hammer."

Sets, Repetitions, Weights: Do three sets of 10 repetitions each. Rest 15 seconds between each set. Use 3-pound dumbbells and go higher as you get stronger.

Triceps: Seated Overhead Press

Develops, shapes, strengthens, and defines the entire triceps, especially the inside and rear heads of this muscle.

Exercise 1

Position: Grasp a dumbbell with an overhead grip, holding it on either side of the ball shape. Sit on a flat bench or chair and raise the dumbbell straight up, locking your elbows and keeping your biceps close to your ears.

Movement: Keeping your biceps close to your head and your elbows stationary, lower the dumbbell in an arc movement by letting your arms descend behind you. Feel a full stretch in your triceps muscle, and without resting and flexing your triceps muscles as you go, return to start position. Willfully flex your triceps muscle and repeat the movement until you have completed your set.

Rest 15 seconds and perform your second set of this exercise. Rest another 15 seconds and perform your third and last set of this exercise.

Rest 15 seconds and repeat the series two more times (nine sets in all). Then move to your next body part, back.

Beware: Your upper arms must remain close to your head throughout the movement. Don't hold your breath. Breathe naturally.

Exercise 2:   Repeat the exercise.

Exercise 3:   Repeat the exercise one last time.

Sets, Repetitions, Weights: Do three sets of 10 repetitions each. Rest 15 seconds between each set. Use 3-pound dumbbells and go higher as you get stronger.

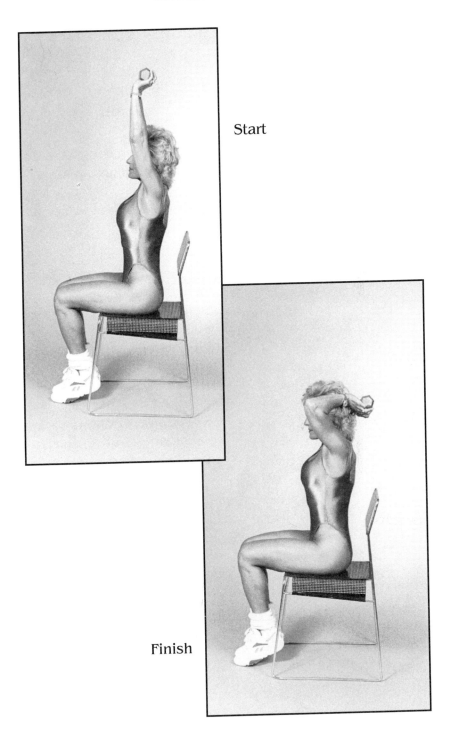

Start

Finish

Back: Double-Arm Bent Row,
Double-Arm Reverse Row

Develops, shapes, strengthens, and defines the back muscles (latissimus dorsi) and helps to develop the biceps.

Exercise 1

Position: Stand with your feet shoulder width apart with a dumbbell held in each hand, palms facing your body. Bend over until your torso is parallel to the floor. Extend your arms straight down and hold the dumbbells in front of your knees.

Movement: Flexing your back muscles as you go, raise the dumbbells up and out to about 6 inches away from the sides of your body, until you cannot go any higher. Willfully flex your back muscles and return to start position. Feel the stretch in your back muscles and repeat the movement until you have completed your set.

Rest 15 seconds and perform your second set of this exercise. Rest another 15 seconds and perform your third and last set of this exercise.

Now move to the next exercise in your back routine, the double-arm reverse row. (Stay in the same exact position, only turn your wrists *out*, palms facing *away* from your body.) Again do three sets as you did here. Then move to the final exercise in your back routine, a repeat of the first exercise, the double-arm bent row, and again do three sets of this exercise.

Congratulations. You have completed your Workout Day 1 workout. The next time you work out you will do your lower body workout, Workout Day 2.

Beware: Don't rise to a near-standing position. Keep your back nearly parallel to the floor throughout the exercise.

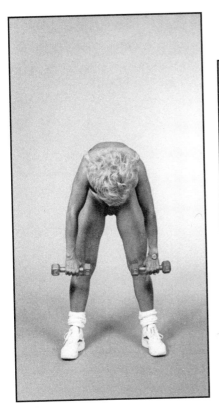

Start

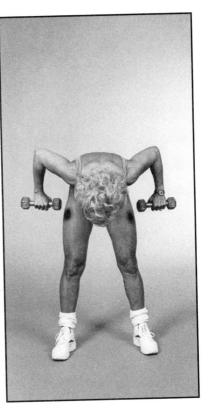

Finish

Exercise 2: Perform this exercise in reverse by facing your palms away from your body, the double-arm reverse row.

Exercise 3: Repeat the first exercise, the double-arm bent row.

Sets, Repetitions, Weights: Do three sets of 10 repetitions each. Rest 15 seconds between each set. Use 3-pound dumbbells and go higher as you get stronger.

WORKOUT DAY 2 LOWER BODY WORKOUT

Thighs: Frog-Leg Front Squat and Regular Squat

This exercise develops, shapes, strengthens, and defines the front and inner thigh.

Exercise 1

Position: Stand with your feet very wide apart and your toes angled outward. Hold a dumbbell in each hand and cross your arms in front of your chest. The ends of the dumbbells should be touching your shoulders. Look straight ahead and keep your back straight.

Movement: Feeling the stretch in your front and inner thigh as you go, descend to a knee bend of about 45 degrees. Without resting and flexing your inner and front thighs as you go, rise to start position. Willfully flex your front and inner thighs and repeat the movement until you have completed your set.

Rest 15 seconds and perform your second set of this exercise. Rest another 15 seconds and perform your third and last set of this exercise.

Now move to the next exercise in your thigh routine, the regular squat. (Simply hold the dumbells down at your sides, palms facing your body.) Again do three sets as you did here. Then move to the final exercise in your thigh routine, a repeat of the first exercise, and again do three sets of this exercise. Then move to your next body part, hip/buttocks.

Beware: Don't drop down or spring back to start position.

Exercise 2: Perform this exercise with feet shoulder width

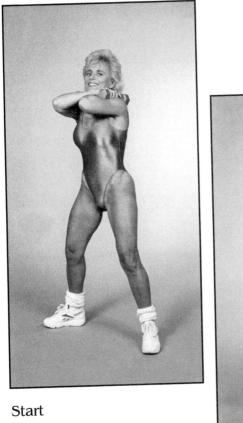

Start

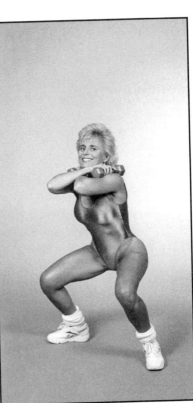

Finish

apart and holding dumbbells straight down at your sides (regular squat).

Exercise 3:   Repeat the first exercise, the frog-leg front squat.

Sets, Repetitions, Weights: Do three sets of 10 repetitions each. Rest 15 seconds between each set. Use 3-pound dumbbells and go higher as you get stronger.

Hip/Buttocks: Prone Butt Lift and Double-Leg Prone Butt Lift

Tightens, tones, shapes, and defines the entire hip/buttocks area, and helps to shape the back thigh muscle and remove saddlebags from the side thigh area.

Exercise 1

Position: Lie on the floor on your stomach, leaning on your elbows for support. Extend your toes behind you, keeping your feet about 12 inches apart.

Movement: Flexing your hip/buttocks muscles and keeping your knees nearly locked, lift one leg until you cannot go any higher. Continuing to keep the pressure on your hip/buttocks area, return to start. Repeat the movement for the other leg. Repeat this alternate movement until you have completed your set.

Rest 15 seconds and perform your second set of this exercise. Rest another 15 seconds and perform your third and last set of this exercise.

Now move to the next exercise in your hip/buttocks routine, the double-leg prone butt lift. (This time you lift both legs at a time. Everything else is the same.) Again do three sets as you did here. Then move to the final exercise in your hip/buttocks routine, a repeat of the first exercise, the prone butt lift, and again do three sets of this exercise. Then move to your next body part, abdominals.

Beware: Don't tense your lower back. Relax as you work.

Exercise 2:   Perform this exercise two legs at a time (double-leg prone butt lift).

Exercise 3:   Repeat the first exercise, the prone butt lift.

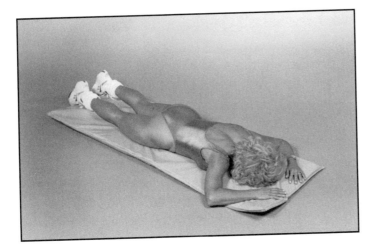

Start

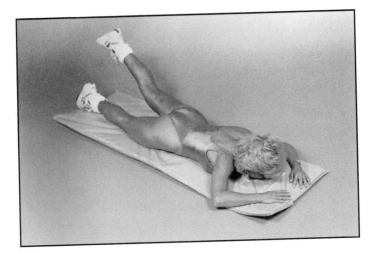

Finish

Sets, Repetitions, Weights: Do three sets of 10 repetitions each. Rest 15 seconds between each set. You do not use weights for the hip/buttocks exercises.

Abdominals: Knee-Raised Crunch and Regular Crunch

Develops, shapes, strengthens, and defines the entire upper abdominal area and helps to strengthen the lower abdominal area.

Exercise 1

Position: Lie flat on your back on the floor and pull your knees up until your legs form an L. You may cross your feet at the ankles. Place your hands behind your head.

Movement: Flexing your entire abdominal area as you go, raise your shoulders off the floor in a curling movement until your shoulders are completely off the floor, all the time keeping your knees raised so that your legs are still in an approximate L shape. Keeping the pressure on your abdominal muscles, return to start and repeat the movement until you have completed your set.

Rest 15 seconds and perform your second set of this exercise. Rest another 15 seconds and perform your third and last set of this exercise.

Now move to the next exercise in your abdominal routine, the regular crunch. (Perform in exactly the same manner, only place soles of feet flat on floor, knees fully bent.) Again do three sets as you did here. Then move to the final exercise in your abdominal routine, a repeat of the first exercise. Again do three sets of this exercise. Then move to your last body part, calves.

Beware: This is exactly the same movement as the crunch, only it is done with the knees raised, so keep them raised and steady.

Exercise 2:   Perform this exercise with your feet flat on the floor, knees bent (regular crunch).

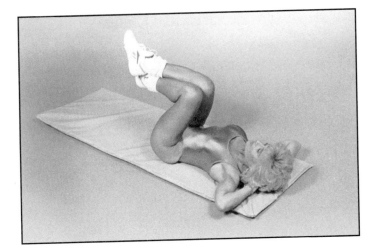

Start

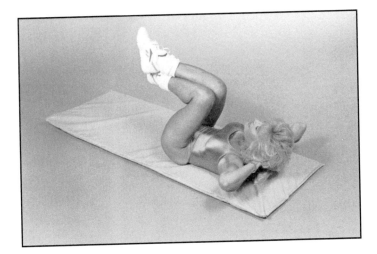

Finish

Exercise 3: Repeat the first exercise, the knee-raised crunch.

Sets, Repetitions, Weights: Do three sets of 10 repetitions each. Rest 15 seconds between each set. You do not use weights for these abdominal exercises.

Calves: Seated Straight-Toe Calf Raise,
Seated Angled-out-Toe Calf Raise,
Seated Angled-in-Toe Calf Raise

Develops, shapes, strengthens, and defines the entire calf muscle (gastrocnemius).

Exercise 1

Position: Sit at the edge of a flat exercise bench or chair with a set of dumbbells held on top of your knees. Plant your heels on the ground.

Movement: Keeping your toes pointed straight ahead and flexing your calf muscles as you go, raise your heels until you cannot go any farther. Willfully flex your calf muscles and return to start position. Feel the stretch in your calf muscles and repeat the movement until you have completed your set.

Rest 15 seconds and perform your second set of this exercise. Rest another 15 seconds and perform your third and last set of this exercise.

Now move to the next exercise in your calf routine, the seated angled-out-toe calf raise. (Do the same way, only angle your toes *out.*) Again do three sets as you did here. Then move to the final exercise in your calf routine, the seated angled-in-toe calf raise. (Do the same way, only angle your toes *in.*) Again do three sets of this exercise.

Congratulations. You have completed your Workout Day 2 workout, the lower body. The next time you work out, you will go back to Workout Day 1, the upper body.

Beware: You have the option of using a thick book if you feel that you are not getting a full range of motion.

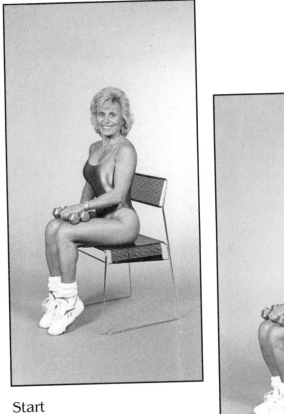

Start

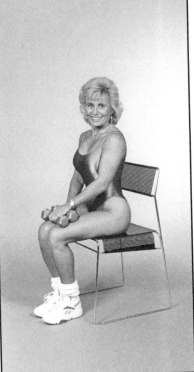

Finish

Exercise 2: Perform this exercise with your toes angled outward.

Exercise 3: Perform this exercise with your toes angled inward.

Sets, Repetitions, Weights: Do three sets of 10 repetitions each. Rest 15 seconds between each set. Use 3-pound dumbbells and go higher as you get stronger.

GOING A STEP FARTHER!

The above workout is meant to be a very simple introductory routine. Chances are you will want a more complete workout, and you may want to choose one that is specifically designed for your needs and goals. Here I give a brief description of each of my exercise books so that you can choose which one may be the best next step for you. But no matter which book you choose, remember that it's a good idea to switch to a different workout every so often. In the past I've said to wait six months before switching, but now I realize that you can switch as early as six weeks if you so desire. If you like a workout, stay with it for three months to a year and then switch.

These books begin with those that take the least time to do to those that take a little longer. Then I explain my specialized book, *The College Dorm Workout.* Finally, I talk about my books addressed specifically to men (although women can do them, too—just as men can use my women's books), *Gut Busters* and *Top Shape.* All books are also listed in the Bibliography.

The 12-Minute Total-Body Workout

This is an excellent workout for those who are complete beginners *and* who have very little time to invest in working out. The only weights you ever use with this workout are 3-pound dumbbells, but you make up for the lower weights by creating your own tension (dynamic tension). Because it involves very light weights, this plan is often used by those who are working around an injury (with the doctor's permission, of course) or who are traveling. The book also explains how to do the workout while traveling and includes detailed information on how to eat in the worst menu situations and still keep to your diet. As the title indicates, the routine takes 12 minutes. It is done six to seven days a week. The main attraction of this workout is its ability to produce muscle hardness. You get very small muscle growth with this workout and you get moderate definition.

Definition: Shape Without Bulk in Fifteen Minutes a Day

This is my most fat-burning workout because you hardly rest at all. As the title indicates, this workout takes 15 minutes a day (there are optional "wonder woman" and "dragon lady" routines that add up to 14 minutes a day). The workout can be done in the traditional split routine, doing one half of the body each workout day, or the full body routine, doing the entire body every other day. (This is the only book I've written that allows working the entire body in one day.) This is accomplished with exercises eliminating one arm (or leg) at a time and adding sets requiring execution of two exercises at a time (the superset). It is the most aerobic of all my workouts and yields the most definition and moderate muscle size. The book has a tear-out wall poster so you don't have to flip pages.

The Fat-Burning Workout

This workout is ideal for those who want to put on a little more muscle than you can with *Definition* but still burn lots of fat, and for those who have a little more time to invest (20 minutes four to six days a week, with additional "intensity" and "insanity" workouts that add up to 20 minutes a day).

The routine requires that three exercises be done at the same time (the "giant set"). This system allows more rests than *Definition*, and hence provides an opportunity for a little more muscle development. Its main attraction is that you can get a near-aerobic workout and burn a great deal of fat while getting significant muscular development.

Bottoms Up!

This book gives a bombs-away workout for those women who need extra work on the hip/butt thigh-stomach area and yet want a total body workout for the upper body, too—with the option of going the extra mile there. The regular routine takes 20 minutes, but there are optional "wild woman" and "terminator" regimens that add up to 20 minutes a workout. It is done four to six days a week.

The system requires that two exercises for different body parts be done at the same time (the "superset between body parts"). It allows you to build slightly more muscle than any other book discussed so far, because it doesn't exhaust the working muscle.

Now or Never

You get a basic workout that will establish a significant muscle base. It requires 1 hour four to six days a week, rather than the 12 to 20 or so minutes required by my other workouts. The reason for the extra time is that longer rests are required between each set because you will be eventually using heavier weights. The workout is ideal not only for those who want to put on a little muscle size but for those who may want to add muscle to only one or two particular body parts—say, for example, your thighs are sagging over your kneecap, and although your other workouts toned the rest of your body just fine, this one area needs more muscle to lift it.

Another important feature of the book is that, in addition to the dumbbell workout, there is a completely illustrated machine workout. Except for *Top Shape*, my other books demonstrate the dumbbell workout and tell which machines to use as a substitute but don't have photographs of the machine workout.

The College Dorm Workout

The book contains not only a workout but a diet for those in the "dorm" situation, where the worst food is served and the space to work out is cramped. The system utilizes the "giant set," as in *The Fat-Burning Workout*, in combination with self-imposed pressure (dynamic tension as used in *The Twelve-Minute Total-Body Workout*). The exercises are specifically designed for those who are forced to work out in cramped quarters. They are done five days a week and take 20 minutes. The workout was invented by my daughter Marthe, after she went off to college and gained 15 pounds. After using the plan to lose the weight and get in shape in eight weeks, she wrote the book so others could benefit, too. This is also a great book for teens and young adults who are not in college.

Although all of my books can be used by either men or women, the books discussed so far are specifically addressed to women. However, I got so many letters from men who were following my women's books that I decided to write two books specifically addressed to their needs.

Gut Busters

I wrote *Gut Busters* because so many men told me, "I think I look good the way I am—except for this gut. If I could only get rid of it." This workout has the seven most effective exercises used by champion bodybuilders to get the "washboard" or "beer can" (not beer belly) abdominals. It's the most intense of all stomach workouts and takes 15 to 20 minutes, six days a week until the ideal stomach is achieved. Then the routine can be done three days a week.

The workout proves beyond a shadow of a doubt that you can "spot change." In other words, a man may have pencil-thin arms, sloping shoulders, and a not-so-great chest, but if he does this stomach workout, he'll have a perfect, rock-hard, ripped stomach. Of course, if he's overweight he must follow the low-fat eating plan in the book or in this book, otherwise the muscles will be covered with fat. Once again I remind you that this workout is equally effective for women.

Top Shape

Similar to *Now or Never*, this workout takes less time: 40 minutes three days a week or 30 minutes four days a week. It has optional "ironman" and "superman" workouts that add up to 15 minutes a workout.

The reason for the reduced time is that men don't have to exercise the hip/buttock area in the same manner as women, who have childbearing hips. In addition, the leg routine for men is optional, since most men are more concerned with their upper body (chest, shoulders, back, arms, and stomach), and feel that their legs are "not so bad" owing to sports activities.

Because so many men like to work in gyms or with home-gym machines, the book gives a complete machine workout in addition to the complete free-weight (dumbbell) workout. And for men who travel, there is an "on the road" routine that covers every situation from most available equipment to no available equipment.

A FINAL WORD

I would love to hear of your progress. Also, if you have any questions regarding the information in this book or in any of my other books—or if you would like to order any of the items on pages 345–346—please write. If you include a stamped, self-addressed envelope, I will answer—but try to keep the letter short and to the point! Your letter will be forwarded to me if you write to:

Joyce Vedral
PO Box 7433-0433
Wantagh, NY 11793-0433

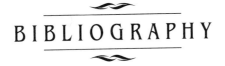

BIBLIOGRAPHY

Joyce Vedral Books

Definition: Shape Without Bulk in Fifteen Minutes a Day. New York: Warner Books, 1995.

Top Shape. New York: Warner Books, 1995.

Bottoms Up! New York: Warner Books, 1993.

Gut Busters. New York: Warner Books, 1992.

The Fat-Burning Workout. New York: Warner Books, 1991.

The 12-Minute Total-Body Workout. New York: Warner Books, 1989.

Now or Never. New York: Warner Books, 1986.

Vedral, Marthe S., and Joyce L. Vedral. *The College Dorm Workout.* New York: Warner Books, 1994.

Self-Help Books

Look In, Look Up, Look Out! Be the Person You Were Meant to Be. New York: Warner Books, 1996 (motivation to stay on target and keep your diet). Also available as a Time Warner Audiobook.

Get Rid of Him. New York: Warner Books, 1993.

Videos

The Bottoms Up Workout: Upper Body. New York: Good Times Video, 1994. $15.98 + $3.00 shipping.

The Bottoms Up Workout: Middle Body. New York: Good Times Video, 1994. $15.98 + $3.00 shipping.

The Bottoms Up Workout: Lower Body. New York: Good Times Video, 1994. $15.98 + $3.00 shipping.

The Fat-Burning Workout, Volume I (The Regular Workout). A-Vision videos. $21.98 + $3.00 shipping.

The Fat-Burning Workout, Volume II (The Intensity and Insanity Workout.) $21.98 + $3.00 shipping.

Other Products

The Joyce Vedral Newsletter. Don't fantasize—*Joycercise!* Share success stories, recipes, questions and answers, motivational tips, inspirational columns, relationship issues, and more. A yearly subscription (4 issues) is $17.98.

Autographed 8x10 color photo. $9.98 + $3.00 shipping.

Videos and other products may be ordered by sending a check or money order to me at P.O. Box 7433, Wantaugh, New York, 11793-0433. Or use this 800 number for credit card orders only: 1-800-879-8244.

Warner Books is not responsible for the delivery or content of the information or materials provided by the author. The reader should address any questions to the author at the above addresss.

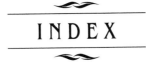

INDEX

348 INDEX